Occupational therapy for adults undergoing total hip replacement

Practice guideline

Second Edition

Royal College of Occupational Therapists

Royal College of Occupational Therapists

Specialist Section
Trauma and Orthopaedics

This publication is endorsed by

British Hip Society

This edition published in 2017
by the Royal College of Occupational Therapists Ltd
106–114 Borough High Street
London SE1 1LB
www.rcot.org.uk

First published in Great Britain in 2012 by the College of Occupational Therapists
This edition supersedes the 2012 edition.

Author: Royal College of Occupational Therapists
Editors: Lauren Porter, Mandy Sainty, Angie Thompson
Guideline Development Review Group: Sheila Harrison, Jamie McNaught, Lauren Porter, Sally Taylor

Original Guideline Development Group: Jade Cope, Christine Gibb, Sheila Harrison, Shirley McCourt, Lauren Porter, Kate Robertson

Category: Practice Guideline
Date for Review: 2022

Other enquires about this document should be addressed to the Royal College of Occupational Therapists Specialist Section – Trauma and Orthopaedics at the above address.

British Library Cataloguing in Publication Data
A catalogue record for this book is available from the British Library

ISBN 978-1-905944-68-2

Typeset by Servis Filmsetting Ltd, Stockport, Cheshire
Digitally printed on demand in Great Britain by the Lavenham Press, Suffolk

MIX
Paper from responsible sources
FSC www.fsc.org
FSC® C010693

Contents

NICE accredited
www.nice.org.uk/accreditation

NICE has renewed accreditation of the process used by the Royal College of Occupational Therapists to produce its practice guidelines. The renewed accreditation is valid until 16 January 2023.

More information on NICE accreditation can be viewed at www.nice.org.uk/accreditation.

This guideline was developed using the processes defined within the *Practice guideline development manual* (College of Occupational Therapists [COT] 2017a).

Readers are referred to the manual to obtain further details of specific stages within the guideline development process, available at:

https://www.rcot.co.uk/practice-resources/rcot-publications/downloads/practice-guideline-development-manual

Foreword (2nd edition)

I am very pleased to have been asked to contribute to the second edition of *Occupational therapy for adults undergoing total hip replacement*. Although it is only five years since the original guidance document was published, the pace of change in healthcare and in particular the field of total hip replacement warrants an update of these guidelines.

Occupational therapy is central to the success of total hip replacement, which is one of the most effective and successful interventions in the whole of medical practice. The success of hip replacement is entirely dependent upon a multidisciplinary team approach, with occupational therapy being a core part of its success.

The updated guidance reflects changes in practice and in particular the requirement for reduction in length of stay. The trend for patients undergoing hip arthroplasty at younger ages continues, as does the increasing numbers of total hip replacements being performed year on year.

National guidance, such as this, is important to disseminate best practice and employ the most effective interventions in the face of potentially diminishing budgets.

On behalf of the British Hip Society I recommend these updated guidelines to you and I am very happy to endorse them on behalf of the Society.

Mr Andrew J Hamer *MD, FRCS (Orth)*
Honorary Secretary
British Hip Society

Foreword (1st edition)

I am delighted to have been asked to write the foreword for *Occupational therapy for adults undergoing total hip replacement*. This guideline is the work of occupational therapists who have had the vision, enthusiasm and perseverance to address this long overdue area; we now have a benchmark of what we should be doing as well as flagging up what we should be improving.

Total hip replacement is a common procedure with statistics continuing to show large numbers of operations being conducted and, indeed, steadily increasing. From 2010–11, over 77,800 primary hip replacements and 9,000 revisions were carried out in England and Wales (National Joint Registry 2011, p35). Yet although the role of occupational therapy is well established and recognised (British Orthopaedic Association 2006), there are rapid changes in the face of practice – not only in the timings of interventions but in the age and range of people needing rehabilitation. Occupational therapists are treating more people of working age who have had hip replacements as well as continuing to treat their more traditional caseload of older patients. They seem to be seeing people earlier, and patients are being discharged more quickly because of the current emphasis on shortening hospital stay and the implementation of 'rapid recovery' initiatives.

Such changes on the coalface are reflected in the widespread variation that exists in national practice. Such variations reflect differences in surgical opinion, in service configurations and the dearth of robust research evidence to underpin clinical practice. This lack of research extends from addressing the most fundamental questions on the use of hip precautions to the best ways of delivering pre-operative and post-operative education and care within a service. Consequently, although this guideline tackles practical issues by examining the literature and making recommendations to guide clinicians, it also highlights the gaps in the evidence. There are key occupational therapy questions to be answered and therapists must rise to this challenge.

Professor Avril Drummond *PhD, MSc, FCOT*
Professor of Healthcare Research and Occupational Therapist
University of Nottingham

Foreword (1st edition)

Following my involvement in the service user consultation for this practice guideline for occupational therapists working with adults undergoing total hip replacement, it is a pleasure to be asked to provide a foreword.

Throughout the development of this guideline service users have been consulted in a meaningful and effective manner, being offered opportunities to share our experiences of undergoing total hip replacement, and we have appreciated clinical staff listening to our views and experiences.

The guideline provides an excellent resource for occupational therapists in the assessment and treatment of people undergoing total hip replacement surgery. It ensures the occupational therapist has the opportunity to gain knowledge of the whole person and that they take into account issues for carers and the service user's mental wellbeing. This, in turn, will benefit the service user by ensuring their care is focused on their recovery and resumption of roles, tailored to their individual needs, and most importantly that they are offered consistent and evidence-based advice and interventions.

Mrs Sue Knowles
Chair, Rushcliffe 50+ Forum Health Sub Group
Nottinghamshire

Key recommendations for implementation

The aim of this practice guideline is to provide specific recommendations that describe the most appropriate care or action to be taken by occupational therapists working with adults undergoing total hip replacement. The recommendations are intended to be used alongside the occupational therapist's clinical expertise and, as such, the clinician is ultimately responsible for the interpretation of this evidence-based guideline in the context of their specific circumstances, environment and service users' needs.

Recommendation statements should not be taken in isolation and must be considered in conjunction with the contextual information provided in this document, together with the details on the strength and quality of the recommendations. The statements are graded based on the Grading of Recommendations Assessment, Development and Evaluation (GRADE) process (Grade Working Group 2004) as described in the Royal College of Occupational Therapists' *Practice guideline development manual 3rd edition* (COT 2017a). The strength of the recommendations is identified via a scoring of 1 (strong) or 2 (conditional), and the quality of the supporting evidence via a grading on a scale of A (high) to D (very low). It is strongly advised that readers study section 11 to understand the guideline methodology, together with the evidence tables in Appendix 7, to be fully aware of the outcome of the literature search and overall available evidence.

Recommendations by category

The recommendation categories reflect six areas of importance for service users undergoing total hip replacement and occupational therapy intervention, and these are presented in the order of prioritisation identified from service user consultation in 2012.

The overall quality of evidence grade reflects the robustness or type of research supporting a recommendation, but not necessarily the recommendation's significance to occupational therapy practice.

Recommendations are identified as being either 'recommended' or 'suggested' (see section 11.5).

'It is recommended. . .' benefits appear to outweigh the risks (or vice versa) for the majority of the target group; most service users would want or should receive this course of intervention or action.

'It is suggested. . .' risks and benefits are more closely balanced, or there is more uncertainty in likely service users' values and preferences; the majority of service users would want this intervention but not all, and therefore they should be supported to arrive at a decision for intervention consistent with the benefits and their values and preferences.

This 2nd edition of the guideline incorporates relevant literature published since 2011. There is one new recommendation. Additionally, some of the 2012 recommendations have been refined to reflect more recent evidence or policy, whilst other statements remain unchanged but supported by further research findings. Annotations are made, where applicable, to reflect the 2017 changes.

Maximised functional independence	
1. ***It is recommended*** that the occupational therapy assessment is comprehensive and considers factors which may affect individual needs, goals, recovery and rehabilitation, including co-morbidities, trauma history, personal circumstances, obesity and pre-operative function. *(Johansson et al 2010 [C]; Lin and Kaplan 2004 [C]; Marks 2008 [C]; Naylor et al 2008 [C]; Ostendorf et al 2004 [C]; Vincent et al 2007 [C]; Vincent et al 2012 [B]; Wang et al 2010 [C])* [New evidence 2017]	1C
2. ***It is recommended*** that goal setting is individualised, enhances realistic expectations of functional independence, and commences at pre-operative assessment. *(Hobbs et al 2011 [C]; Judge et al 2011 [C]; Mancuso et al 2003 [C])* [New evidence 2017]	1C
3. ***It is recommended*** that occupational therapists ensure that they provide clear communication and advice that is consistent with that of other members of the multidisciplinary team. *(Drummond et al 2013 [C]; Fielden et al 2003 [C])* [New evidence 2017]	1C
4. ***It is recommended*** that depression and anxiety status are taken into account during pre-operative and post-operative intervention due to their potential for impact on recovery. *(Caracciolo and Giaquinto 2005 [C]; Nickinson et al 2009 [C])*	1C
5. ***It is recommended*** that cognitive status is taken into account during pre-operative and post-operative intervention due to its potential for impact on recovery. *(Wang and Emery 2002 [C]; Wong et al 2002 [C])*	1C
6. ***It is recommended*** that service users are fully involved in decisions about the equipment required to enable them to carry out daily living activities and to comply with any hip precautions in their home environment post-surgery. *(Thomas et al 2010 [D])*	1D
7. ***It is recommended*** that service users are given advice on effective pain management strategies, to decrease pre-operative pain experience and sleep disturbance, and enhance post-operative physical function. *(Berge et al 2004 [B]; Montin et al 2007 [C]; Parsons et al 2009 [C])*	1B

8.	***It is suggested*** that standardised assessment and outcome measures are used, where appropriate, to determine functional outcomes and occupational performance in rehabilitation settings, either inpatient or community based. *(Alviar et al 2011 [B]; Gillen et al 2007 [C]; Kiefer and Emery 2004 [C]; Oberg et al 2005 [D])* [New evidence 2017]	2C

Reduced anxiety		
9.	***It is recommended*** that the pre-operative assessment undertaken by the occupational therapist allows adequate time for individualised questions and discussion of expectations and anxieties. *(Fielden et al 2003 [C]; McDonald et al 2014 [A]; McDonald et al 2004 [A]; Montin et al 2007 [C])* [New evidence 2017]	1A
10.	***It is suggested*** that occupational therapists offer support and advice to service users who may be anxious about an accelerated discharge home. *(Heine et al 2004 [D]; Hunt et al 2009 [D]; Montin et al 2007 [C])*	2C
11.	***It is recommended*** that pre-operative assessment and education is carried out in the most appropriate environment for the service user. For the majority of service users a clinic environment is appropriate, but where needs are complex, a home assessment should be an available option. *(Crowe and Henderson 2003 [B]; Drummond et al 2012 [C]; Orpen and Harris 2010 [C]; Rivard et al 2003 [B])*	1B
12.	***It is suggested*** that provision of equipment pre-operatively may facilitate familiarity and confidence in use. *(Fielden et al 2003 [C]; Orpen and Harris 2010 [C])*	2C
13.	***It is suggested*** that service users may value being treated by the same occupational therapist throughout the process, from pre-operative assessment/education to post-operative rehabilitation wherever possible. *(Spalding 2003 [C])*	2C
14.	***It is suggested*** that occupational therapists should contribute to standardised pre-operative education interventions, providing information, advice and demonstrations where relevant (e.g. of joint protection principles, equipment). *(Coudeyre et al 2007 [B]; Johansson et al 2007 [B]; Spalding 2003 [C]; Spalding 2004 [C]; Soever et al 2010 [C])*	2B

Resumption of meaningful occupation	
15. ***It is recommended*** that work roles are discussed at the earliest opportunity as part of a comprehensive assessment. *(Bohm 2010 [C]; Cowie et al 2013 [C]; Malviya et al 2014 [A]; Mobasheri et al 2006 [D]; Nunley et al 2011 [C]; Sankar et al 2013 [C])* [New evidence 2017]	1C
16. ***It is suggested*** that for service users who are working, advice is provided relating to maintaining their work role pre-operatively, post-operative expectations and relevant information for employers. *(Bohm 2010 [C]; Cowie et al 2013 [C]; Malviya et al 2014 [A]; Mobasheri et al 2006 [D]; Nunley et al 2011 [C]; Parsons et al 2009 [D]; Sankar et al 2013 [C])* [New evidence 2017]	2C
17. ***It is recommended*** that occupational therapists provide advice to facilitate service users to establish previous and new roles and relationships, and shift their focus from disability to ability. *(Grant et al 2009 [C]; McHugh and Luker 2012 [C])* [New evidence 2017]	1C
18. ***It is recommended*** that occupational therapists encourage early discussion and goal setting for community reintegration. *(de Groot et al 2008 [D]; Gillen et al 2007 [C]; Heiberg et al 2013 [D]; McHugh and Luker 2012 [C]; Smith et al 2015 [B])* [Statement amended, new evidence 2017]	1C
19. ***It is suggested*** that the return to physical and sporting activities is considered within an occupational therapy assessment and interventions. *(Abe et al 2014 [C]; Cowie et al 2013 [C]; Harding et al 2014 [C]; Ollivier et al 2014 [C]; Vissers et al 2013 [C]; Wagenmakers et al 2011 [C]; Williams et al 2012 [C]; Wilson and Villar 2011 [D])* [New statement and evidence 2017]	2C
20. ***It is suggested*** that where specific needs are identified, the occupational therapist refers the service user on to community rehabilitation, reablement or intermediate care services to enhance community reintegration. *(de Groot et al 2008 [D]; Gillen et al 2007 [C])*	2C

Hip precautions	
21. ***It is recommended*** that occupational therapists consult with the surgical team regarding any specific precautions to be followed post-operatively. *(Barnsley et al 2015 [B]; Hol et al 2010 [B]; McQuaid et al 2014 [C]; Peak et al 2005 [B]; Restrepo et al 2011 [B]; Smith et al 2016 [A]; Stewart and McMillan 2011 [C]; van der Weegen et al 2016 [B]; Ververeli et al 2009 [B])* [New evidence 2017]	1B

22. ***It is recommended*** that occupational therapists advise service users, where protocol includes precautions, on appropriate position behaviours for those daily activities applicable to the individual's needs, ranging from getting in/out of a car to answering the telephone. *(Coole et al 2013 [C]; Drummond et al 2012 [C]; Malik et al 2002 [D]; Peak et al 2005 [B]; Smith and Sackley 2016 [C]; Stewart and McMillan 2011 [C]; Ververeli et al 2009 [B])* [New evidence 2017]	1B
23. ***It is suggested*** that given the increase in evidence of improved service user satisfaction and earlier functional independence, without adverse effects on dislocation rates when hip precautions are relaxed or discontinued, occupational therapists engage in local discussion/review of hip precaution protocols with their surgical and multidisciplinary teams. *(Barnsley et al 2015 [B]; Coole et al 2013 [C]; Drummond et al 2012 [C]; McQuaid et al 2014 [C]; O'Donnell et al 2006 [D]; Peak et al 2005 [B]; Restrepo et al 2011 [B]; Smith and Sackley 2016 [C]; Smith et al 2016 [A]; van der Weegen et al 2016 [B]; Ververeli et al 2009 [B])* [Statement amended, new evidence 2017]	2B

Enhanced recovery	
24. ***It is recommended*** that occupational therapists optimise length of stay, with due reference to care pathways and enhanced recovery programme guidance. *(Arshad et al 2014 [C]; Berend et al 2004 [C]; Bottros et al 2010 [C]; Brunenberg et al 2005 [C]; Husted et al 2008 [C]; Ibrahim et al 2013 [B]; Kim et al 2003 [B])* [New evidence 2017]	1B
25. ***It is recommended*** that the occupational therapist is involved in early multidisciplinary post-operative intervention for service users following hip replacement, providing either inpatient or home-based rehabilitation. *(Aasvang et al 2015 [D]; Ibrahim et al 2013 [B]; Iyengar et al 2007 [C]; Khan et al 2008 [A]; Pape et al 2013 [C]; Siggeirsdottir et al 2005 [C])* [New evidence 2017]	1A

Reduced demand on support services	
26. ***It is suggested*** that there are potential benefits in including informal carers in pre-operative assessment/education, and post-operative intervention, to maximise service user independence and reduce carer stress. *(Chow 2001 [C])*	2C

It is additionally recommended that occupational therapists use the audit tool that is available to support this guideline (see section 8) to audit against the above recommendations.

1 Introduction

Total hip replacement has been identified as an effective treatment for the hip joint that causes pain and functional impairment where conservative management is no longer effective. Indications for a primary total hip replacement are pain and disability arising from osteoarthritis or inflammatory arthritis in the hip joint (British Orthopaedic Association [BOA] 2012).

The National Institute for Health and Care Excellence [NICE] Clinical Guideline *Osteoarthritis: care and management* recommends that clinicians should:

> *Consider referral for joint replacement surgery for people with osteoarthritis who experience joint symptoms (pain, stiffness and reduced function) that have a substantial impact on their quality of life and are refractory to non-surgical treatment. Refer for consideration of joint surgery before there is prolonged and established functional limitation and severe pain.* (NICE 2014, p18)

Outcomes include improved symptoms and functional status with continuation in improvement for the first year after the operation (Royal College of Surgeons of England; BOA 2000, p8).

Hip replacement may also be indicated following trauma to the hip, such as in hip fracture, being particularly relevant for adults with pre-existing joint disease, medium/high activity levels, and who are not cognitively impaired (NICE 2011, Scottish Intercollegiate Guidelines Network [SIGN] 2009).

This practice guideline focuses on total hip replacement, completed as primary or revision elective surgery, or following trauma. It is recognised that some of the recommendations will be directly applicable to elective surgery only, rather than trauma surgery, and also that occupational therapists treating service users undergoing two-stage revision surgery will need to follow local protocols and post-operative instructions. However, the majority of the recommendations will be appropriate to service users undergoing a total hip replacement whatever the pre-disposing circumstances.

Occupational therapy staff involved in treating service users post hip fracture should, however, also refer to national hip fracture guidelines (SIGN 2009, NICE 2011) and the quality standard (NICE 2012), together with national falls guidelines (NICE 2013) and professional practice guidelines on the prevention and management of falls (COT 2015a).

1.1 Practice requirement for the guideline

Occupational therapy is a key intervention for individuals receiving a total hip replacement, as identified within the British Orthopaedic Association good practice guidance (BOA 2012), and in national orthopaedic and musculoskeletal programmes, frameworks and audits (Wales Audit Office 2015, Department of Health 2006, National Audit Office [NAO] 2003).

The number of occupational therapists specifically working across the care pathway with adults who have osteoarthritis or who receive a total hip replacement is not known. However, given the number of hip replacements across the four countries of the United Kingdom (UK), it is predicted that a considerable proportion of the 36,217 occupational therapists registered with the Health and Care Professions Council (HCPC 2016a) may come into contact with service users receiving a hip replacement at some stage during their health or social care intervention. A UK national survey of orthopaedic occupational therapists reported that the mean percentage of department/service resources used to support service users receiving a total hip replacement was 39%. It also indicated that on average, an excess of two hours was spent in face-to-face contact, and over one hour in non-direct contact (Drummond et al 2012).

Known evidence from both the literature (Smith and Sackley 2016, Coole et al 2013, Drummond et al 2012) and expert practitioners involved in the Royal College of Occupational Therapists Specialist Section – Trauma and Orthopaedics confirms that differences exist in practice across the UK in areas which include pre-operative assessment and education processes, use of hip precautions and equipment provision. Prior to the publication of the first edition of this guideline in 2012, there had been no formal national guidance for occupational therapists working with service users who had received a total hip replacement.

The number of service users undergoing total hip replacement in the UK is high and expected to increase (Culliford et al 2015). This demand for orthopaedic services, combined with the pressures of waiting list management, means there is a constant drive for improved efficiency in service provision. In this context, and with the significant variation in practice across the UK, this practice guideline for occupational therapy and total hip replacement aims to assist clinicians and managers in achieving the best possible outcomes for the service user, utilising resources in line with evidence and best practice.

1.2 Topic identification process

Total hip replacement, as a guideline development topic, was identified by the Royal College of Occupational Therapists Specialist Section – Trauma and Orthopaedics (RCOTSS – Trauma and Orthopaedics).

A decision was made to focus the guideline on total hip replacement both as an elective procedure and following trauma (i.e. fractured neck of femur). While it is recognised that there are differences for the service user having elective compared with trauma surgery, the role of the occupational therapist and the care pathway will have many similarities. The decision was made not to expand the guideline further to include other types of surgery following hip fracture (such as hemiarthroplasty) as it was felt this was addressed in other available national clinical guidelines (SIGN 2009, NICE 2011).

A proposal to produce a practice guideline for occupational therapy within the field of total hip replacement was developed by the RCOTSS – Trauma and Orthopaedics, and this was subsequently approved by the Royal College of Occupational Therapists' Practice Publications Group in March 2011.

1.3 National context: hip replacement statistics

Information on hip replacement procedures in the UK is recorded; however, the data is not available as a single source.

The National Joint Registry holds details on joint replacement surgery for England, Wales and Northern Ireland, and includes procedures undertaken by both the National Health Service and the independent healthcare sector. In Scotland, the Scottish Arthroplasty Project uses Scottish Morbidity Records sent by hospitals to the Information Services Division to ascertain the number and outcome of joint replacements undertaken.

Table 1: UK primary hip joint procedure statistics

	England	Wales	Northern Ireland	Scotland
Primary hip joint procedures (numbers)	83,213	3,925	2,150	7,907
Year	2015	2015	2015	2015
Average age		69		67
Percentage female		59.8%		59.4%
Percentage male		40.2%		40.6%
Source	National Joint Registry (2016)			NHS National Services Scotland (2016)

The numbers of primary hip joint replacements completed have been increasing. In England and Wales, for example, an additional 9,338 procedures were reported in the 2016 National Joint Registry Report compared with the 2011 report (National Joint Registry 2011). Scotland has also seen an increase, with an additional 739 procedures recorded in the 2016 report compared with the 2010 report (NHS National Services Scotland 2010).

The statistics demonstrate that there is a high volume of service users in the UK undergoing primary total hip replacement, with these numbers continuing to rise on an annual basis.

1.4 Context of service delivery

The *NICE musculoskeletal conditions overview* includes a number of components, such as pathways for arthritis and for trauma, both of which include total hip replacement as a management option. The pathway provides reference to associated clinical guidelines (NICE 2017).

The Musculoskeletal Services Framework (Department of Health [DH] 2006), which was endorsed by the Royal College of Occupational Therapists, focused on best practice guidance to support people with musculoskeletal conditions, whether a result of disease, injury or development disorder. It was intended to assist in the delivery of improved access for service users, and in the reduction of waiting times for treatment. While directly applicable to England, the vision is one which can still be universally shared by all occupational therapists working in this field of practice:

> *The vision is that people with musculoskeletal conditions can access high-quality, effective and timely advice, assessment, diagnosis and treatment to enable them to fulfil their optimum health potential and remain independent.* (DH 2006, p6)

The framework included a pathway for adults with hip pain, demonstrating the service user flow from pain onset to surgery.

The NHS Wales National Orthopaedic Programme – Delivery Framework (Wales Audit Office 2015, p59) is comparable in terms of identifying the involvement of occupational therapists throughout the pathway. Occupational therapists should be involved in active management within primary healthcare teams in the community, in musculoskeletal clinics and in hospital services. Key within this is the multi-professional pre-operative assessment with identification of potential post-operative service user concerns, the provision of adaptive equipment, and discharge planning to prevent discharge delays following surgery.

Multidisciplinary working and 'shared care' are seen as being fundamental to the approach, together with integrated care pathways based on the entire journey taken by a service user.

The importance of an agreed process for continued rehabilitation and evidence-based follow-up where indicated are also identified as part of the flow process. It is therefore important that total hip replacement elective surgery and the guideline recommendations within this publication are seen in the context of a wider clinical pathway.

The involvement of occupational therapists, particularly in pre-operative assessment, is also highlighted in the consensus document, *Primary total hip replacement: a guide to good practice*, published by the British Orthopaedic Association (BOA 2012). It states that the involvement of occupational therapists, along with other members of the multidisciplinary team, can assist in preventing cancellation of surgery, allow co-morbidities and risk factors to be identified, and facilitate discharge planning. The home circumstances and availability of carers after discharge from hospital are also identified as being important (BOA 2012, p9). Pre-admission assessment provides an opportunity for service user education and establishing expectations, particularly with regard to the risk and benefits of the operation and the discussion of goals (BOA 2012, p9).

The period between admission and discharge for routine elective surgery has reduced in recent years, with a median length of stay recorded as four days for a cemented total hip replacement and three days for an uncemented total hip replacement in England during 2014/2015 (NHS Digital 2015). In Scotland the average length of stay in 2015 was reported as 5.1 days (NHS National Services Scotland 2016). Length of stay is associated with cost, and there is an expectation that clinical pathways in addition to promoting best practice will reduce length of stay and shorten post-operative rehabilitation.

Sourcing information on an indicative cost of elective hip replacement intervention across the UK is not simple. It is complicated by the different funding and payment structures within each country, and the variables in the nature of service delivery. To provide a proxy indicator of the cost of a total hip replacement for this guideline, the *2016/17 National Prices and National Tariff Workbook* for England (where the majority of hip replacements are undertaken) has therefore been used (Monitor and NHS England 2016a). This defines a primary total hip replacement best practice tariff of £5,150 where no complications or co-morbidities exist (the figure is increased to £5,884 where complications and co-morbidities are identified).

Best practice tariffs have been applied to elective total hip replacements in England from 2011–2012, demonstrating how clinical pathways can be potentially linked with cost.

Best practice tariffs target interventions with high impact and a strong evidence base or clinical consensus of best practice characteristics. The purpose of the best practice tariff for primary hip replacements is to link payment to the outcomes that are important from the service user's perspective, and aim to reduce the unexplained variation between providers in the outcomes reported by service users. The use of the Patient Reported Outcome Measures (PROMs) is key to this approach. Information is collected about a service user's health status (or health-related quality of life) before surgery, and again six months after the procedure, with any change in health state attributed to the intervention (assessed using the case mix adjusted condition-specific Oxford Hip Score for primary joint replacements only). Reporting to the National Joint Registry is also a requirement (Monitor and NHS England 2016b, p64). The national tariff payment system also identifies the pathway for post-discharge activity for primary non-trauma total hip replacements as including one occupational therapy appointment (Monitor and NHS England 2016b, p13).

In terms of best practice approaches to intervention, 'enhanced recovery' (or rapid recovery) programmes provide a more 'front-loaded pathway' to ensure aspects of recuperation and social care are addressed pre-operatively to reduce delays post-operatively (i.e. by pre-operative equipment provision). The goal of these programmes is to achieve an improved service user experience by virtue of the service user being more informed. In some localities 'joint schools' operate, consisting of a multidisciplinary education session in which the service user is provided with the relevant information and encouraged to bring along a 'coach' (family member or friend) to assist and support them (Worrall 2010). Enhanced recovery programmes can also lead to a more streamlined approach to care and shorter length of stay (NHS South East Coast 2012).

Empowering the service user with information can be effective in assisting with motivation and developing appropriate expectations about achievements along the pathway. The need for effective pre-operative assessment and provisional discharge planning is, therefore, imperative.

2 The occupational therapy role

Occupational therapy involvement with adults undergoing a total hip replacement takes place in the acute inpatient or pre-operative setting, although not exclusively (Drummond et al 2012). Given the wider context of the 'service user flow', it is, therefore, important to draw attention to the person-centred and holistic philosophy of occupational therapy.

> *Occupational therapy enables people to achieve health, wellbeing and life satisfaction through participation in occupation.* (WFOT 2013, p48)
>
> *'Occupation' refers to practical and purposeful activities that allow people to live independently and have a sense of identity. This could be essential day-to-day tasks such as self-care, work or leisure.* (COT 2016)

Clinical reasoning must take account of individual preferences and needs, including the complexities of treating service users with multiple pathologies, or those with cognitive or emotional dysfunctions, dementia and learning disabilities.

Shorter length of hospital stay has necessitated, in many services, prioritisation of inpatient therapy to elements such as mobility and self-care that are essential for safe discharge, rather than adopting a more holistic stance. Occupational therapy recognises that service users have a wide range and diversity of goals, specific to their own situation. Part of the remit of the hospital-based occupational therapist, therefore, includes signposting and referral to community teams, in recognition that not all needs may be addressed within the hospital environment. This may be due to service user functional readiness and restricted resources, and the fact that some needs related to roles and occupations may be more appropriately responded to within the service user's usual home environment. It is also anticipated that by empowering service users to understand principles of safe movement, fatigue management and graded return to activity, they can, as an 'expert service user', apply these principles to tasks within their individual lifestyle, returning to meaningful activity as soon as possible following surgery.

Assessment prior to surgery provides an opportunity for the service user to discuss their goals and desired outcomes with the occupational therapist. The timing of that assessment varies nationally, although the majority of service users awaiting a hip replacement are usually seen about four weeks prior to surgery (Drummond et al 2012). The assessment may include discussion of any concerns or anxieties the service user may have regarding their current functional abilities in relation to self-care, productivity and leisure, within the context of their roles, occupations and environment. Drummond et al (2012) identified within a national survey that those daily living activities most commonly discussed with service users are kitchen activities, bath or shower transfers, car transfers, strip washing and dressing techniques. Activities most practised are bed, chair and toilet transfers, followed by dressing practice. Assessment needs to be sensitive and mindful of the cognitive functioning of the service user, and delivery of all stages of intervention adapted accordingly. Goals can then be developed and a treatment plan jointly agreed.

The home situation is discussed from the perspective that the service user is expert in this domain and their specific needs and choices. The service user can inform the occupational therapist about specific heights of their furniture (chair, bed and toilet) so that equipment may be prescribed to compensate for lack of function, or to enable activities to be continued while observing hip precautions that restrict certain movements (should this be required by team protocols). The general layout of the home, position of bathroom and toilet, and any potential areas of difficulty, such as steep stairs or difficult access, can be identified by the service user and discussed with the occupational therapist in order to jointly plan agreed intervention. Where an individual has an established condition and is awaiting elective surgery, they may have already been provided with equipment to assist them in daily activities. The most common item prescribed by occupational therapists for service users receiving a primary total hip replacement is a raised toilet seat, with the other most frequently prescribed items being chair and bed raisers, perching stools, long-handled reachers and dressing aids (Drummond et al 2012).

The service user also has an opportunity to discuss issues relating to support which may be needed on discharge. This can identify if a care package could be beneficial, or whether they have arranged support from family and friends or private providers. Equally, some service users may be carers or parents and thus have responsibility for others. This stage of the intervention may take the form of a discussion with the service user, completion of a form by the service user/family, or a visit to the service user's home.

Education to build on a service user's current knowledge, address concerns and provide an opportunity to discuss what their surgery will involve and how recovery will impact on their daily lives is an important element of pre-operative occupational therapy.

Education may be delivered individually or as a group teaching session. Group sessions may be delivered in a 'joint school' incorporating information from the consultant (regarding the procedure) and anaesthetist, in addition to teaching and facilitation by other members of the multidisciplinary team. This will commonly include information on any hip precaution protocols in place to reduce the risk of dislocation.

Accessible information which can assist in improving health literacy is essential and it may be necessary to provide easy read information, or use other adapted forms of communication, for service users with additional needs. With the advance of technology there is also the opportunity to consider other options, which could increase service user choice about how they access information, such as websites/mobile apps or digital television.

Empowering the service user to take responsibility for their own health management is important, as it is believed that 'expert service users' will be more involved in their care and outcomes, leading to increased reablement following surgery.

Hip precautions, which are restrictions on range of movement and activities undertaken by the service user, were traditionally implemented as a preventative measure. The aim was to reduce the likelihood of dislocation by facilitating the healing of soft tissues surrounding the replaced hip (Restrepo et al 2011).

Variations exist in clinicians' views (Coole et al 2013, Smith and Sackley 2016) and in practice; some services now have no routine hip precautions, but where they exist, these generally advise not to flex the hip beyond 90 degrees, and to avoid adduction and rotation of the hip. Risk of dislocation can be influenced by factors such as surgical approach and whether surgery is completed electively or post-trauma. Weight-bearing restrictions may also be in place. There is disparity in the length of time to which it is recommended that precautions should be adhered, but this is usually between six weeks and three months, as directed by the surgeon (this can vary from surgeon to surgeon within the same department).

As more evidence becomes available to challenge the efficacy of hip precautions, this is an area of practice likely to see ongoing change, and occupational therapists should, therefore, take this into account when implementing the recommendations in this practice guideline.

The service user story

"I was very impressed with the support I received from the occupational therapists when I was in hospital in January 2011. From the outset, their approach was pro-active and very soon after arriving at the hospital there was a group meeting with a member of the department. The purpose of this was to prepare us (pre-operation) for the pitfalls (post-operation) and how to avoid these. The do's and don'ts were explained to us, we were shown how to dress, what aids we would have and how these could be used. This meeting helped to relieve anxiety and allowed us to prepare both mentally and physically for how we could cope post-operation. After hip surgery there were further individual meetings with occupational therapists, where I had to demonstrate my ability to dress as taught. I was also taken to the 'home area', to be shown how best I should move around the kitchen once home. After this demonstration, I was then observed putting this into practice. Before my discharge from hospital I had also to demonstrate that I could manage stairs using sticks/crutches as I had been taught. All the aids to support me at home had been supplied prior to my stay in hospital. However, the commodes had not been adjusted/fitted. In the hospital, my partner was given a very helpful demonstration by the occupational therapist so that he was able to adjust the equipment to suit me for my return home. All in all, I had an excellent experience as a patient at the Golden Jubilee and I am very grateful for the part the occupational therapists played in that experience. What impressed me most was the teamwork displayed not only with the occupational therapy department, but across all the departments/groups involved in my care. Nurses, surgical team, doctors, occupational therapists, physiotherapists, auxiliaries, cleaning staff – everyone seemed to know what part he/she had to play, when it was to be played and how in terms of patient care. This close working together made for efficiency and a high standard of care – all of which reduced anxiety for me and made me feel confident about my outcomes post-operation. . . . Forgot to say how useful the brochure 'Patient Guide to Hips' was in preparing me pre- and post-surgery. Practised exercises pre-op, which made it easier post-op."

Golden Jubilee National Hospital service user feedback (2012)

3 Objective of the guideline

The guideline objective:

To describe the most appropriate care or action to be taken by occupational therapists working with adults undergoing total hip replacement.

The objective addresses occupational therapy intervention during the service user's journey along the total hip replacement pathway with reference to:

- Pre-operative education and intervention (for elective cases).
- The inpatient episode of care and rehabilitation following surgery.
- Care in the community following discharge from the inpatient setting (including rehabilitation and reablement).

It is intended that occupational therapists use this guideline to inform their work with service users, with a particular focus on empowering the service user to be fully engaged and take responsibility for their recovery from surgery and achieving individual goals.

This guideline should be used in conjunction with the current versions of the following professional practice requirements, of which knowledge and adherence are assumed:

- *Standards of conduct, performance and ethics* (Health and Care Professions Council 2016b).
- *Standards of proficiency – occupational therapists* (Health and Care Professions Council 2013).
- *Code of Ethics and Professional Conduct* (College of Occupational Therapists 2015b).
- *Professional standards for occupational therapy practice* (College of Occupational Therapists 2017b).

It is intended that this guideline be used alongside the therapist's clinical expertise and, as such, the clinician is ultimately responsible for the interpretation of the evidence-based recommendations in the context of their specific circumstances and the service user's individual needs.

4 Guideline scope

4.1 Clinical question

The key question covered by this guideline is:

What evidence is there to support occupational therapy intervention with adults over the age of 18 undergoing total hip replacement?

The expert practitioners within the guideline development group identified, from their knowledge of the evidence base and own clinical expertise, that occupational therapy intervention with adults undergoing a total hip replacement in practice includes a number of clinical, health and social care areas:

- Service user engagement (i.e. empowering the service user to be responsible for their rehabilitation through education, setting and prioritisation of rehabilitation goals).
- Performance of activities of daily living (personal, domestic and community tasks); for example, discussing adaptation of tasks and practising completion of tasks using new techniques. Tasks may include getting washed and dressed, meal preparation, laundry, shopping or other activities identified by the service user.
- Post-operative functional mobility and transfers – practising walking with mobility aids, step and stair negotiation, transfers on/off bed, chair, toilet, in/out of car, etc., in line with any recommended movement precautions.
- Pre- and post-operative cognitive and emotional function and impact on occupational performance are taken into account during all stages of assessment and intervention or action, and techniques adapted or strategies employed as required.
- Environmental considerations (i.e. ensuring safe home environment for discharge, which may involve discussions with the service user regarding current set-up, access visits, home visits).
- Social considerations (i.e. ensuring adequate support in the community and liaising with the service user, informal carers and health and social care services as required).
- Work and leisure activities (i.e. discussion regarding adapting tasks and environment to suit the service user and maximise functional independence in both the pre- and post-operative phase, including appropriate travel arrangements and return to driving).
- Return to previous roles (i.e. discussion regarding adapting activities and environment to empower the service user to resume meaningful roles such as spouse/partner [including sexual relations], family member, caregiver, worker, community member).
- Comprehensive falls assessment (where the service user has sustained a hip fracture as a result of a fall), with interventions targeted towards modifiable risk factors (NICE 2013).

Individual service user goals are identified at the assessment stage. These are highly influential on intervention following total hip replacement, when they will be discussed between the occupational therapist and the service user and prioritised accordingly.

It is recognised that the occupational therapist works as part of a multidisciplinary team, and that there are some key areas above that overlap with the role of other healthcare professionals working with the group of service users. These include but are not limited to:

- Personal activities of daily living, also addressed by nursing staff.
- Functional mobility and transfers, also addressed by physiotherapists.
- Social considerations and return to previous roles, also addressed by social workers.

Occupational therapy staff must work alongside these professionals in accordance with local service arrangements to ensure the needs of the service user are met.

Intervention must be compatible with desired outcomes for the service user, and this person-centred perspective underpins occupational therapy practice.

The guideline development group members identified some key outcomes of occupational therapy intervention. These were categorised as service user-centred or service delivery-centred:

Service user-centred outcomes:

- Reduced anxiety.
- Maximised functional independence.
- Reintegration into the community.
- Resumption of roles.

Service delivery-centred outcomes:

- Reduced demand on support services.
- Enhanced recovery (referred to as 'decreased length of hospital stay' in the first edition).
- Low readmission rates.

It can be difficult to determine the importance of specific outcomes to individual service users, particularly as in occupational therapy those outcomes are frequently interdependent. A core part of the service user involvement in this guideline development project was to review and judge the importance of these outcomes from the service user perspective (section 10.3).

4.2 Target population

This practice guideline relates to adults receiving a total hip replacement. To further define the target population:

- Adults are defined as any person aged 18 years and over.
- There are no restrictions/limitations on gender, ethnicity or cultural background.
- The condition covered by this guideline includes all types of implant/prosthesis and total hip replacement surgical approaches (such as the anterolateral approach,

posterolateral approach, minimally invasive approach), and the application of enhanced recovery principles.

- The guideline recommendations should be considered for adults undergoing total hip replacement as an elective procedure (primary or revision) or following trauma. It is recognised, however, that some recommendations (e.g. those focusing on pre-operative assessment and intervention) will not be applicable for those undergoing the procedure following trauma, and also that in the instance of complex two-stage revision surgery local policies and post-operative recommendations may need to be taken into account. Professional judgement should therefore be exercised for appropriate application of these guidelines.
- Occupational therapists should take into account potential health inequalities and any social determinants of health that may be appropriate to the provision of services (Marmot et al 2010, p15). There are no exclusions for co-morbidities; however, each service user should be assessed individually (taking into account relevant co-morbidities) when determining appropriate care or action in relation to the guideline recommendations.

There are no populations or sub-groups that are not covered by this guideline other than those less than 18 years of age.

4.3 Target audience

This practice guideline's principal audience is occupational therapists working with adults undergoing total hip replacement. It is, therefore, primarily relevant to occupational therapists who come into contact with this group of service users as they progress through the care pathway for total hip replacement, from pre-operative preparation, to inpatient rehabilitation, and on to community care following discharge from hospital.

For that reason, this guideline will be applicable in many settings: community/outpatient clinics, the service user's home, acute or community hospitals. The publication will be useful to occupational therapists working in health, as well as social services. It can be applied to National Health Service (NHS) settings, as well as the independent sector.

In addition to occupational therapy staff, it is suggested that this practice guideline will be relevant:

- To members of the multidisciplinary team; for example, physiotherapists, nursing staff, social workers, healthcare assistants and surgeons. This guideline may facilitate a better understanding of the role of the occupational therapist in total hip replacement. This could lead to better working between disciplines, with improved outcomes for service users.
- As an educational tool, orientating individuals to the occupational therapy role in total hip replacement (e.g. may be utilised by occupational therapy students, technical instructors, support workers and assistants).
- For social care providers who would also benefit from reviewing this document to support interdisciplinary working, facilitating a safe and effective discharge and transition back into the community for the service user.
- As evidence for managers and commissioners within healthcare services of the valuable role of occupational therapy with this service user group, and may be used as a reference tool to justify staffing levels, funding, etc.

- For private providers/independent sector (i.e. private discharge schemes) to specifically tailor service provision/staffing to suit this group of service users.
- To equipment providers/trusted assessors, who would also benefit from reviewing this document to better understand the needs of this specific group of service users.
- To service users themselves and their carers. The guideline has the potential to enable them to be better informed about the occupational therapy process, supporting the development of the service user as an 'expert'. Service users will also be more aware of models of service delivery that do not meet agreed evidence-based practice, enhancing their potential to contribute to quality improvements.

It is intended that this guideline provides a comprehensive evidence-based resource for occupational therapists working with adults undergoing total hip replacement, as well as an informative document for the wider audience identified above.

5 Background to clinical condition

A person may require a total hip replacement due to underlying disease to the joint (usually involving a planned, elective admission), or as a result of a traumatic injury. The most common indication for having a total hip replacement is osteoarthritis. Other causes may include rheumatoid arthritis (a chronic inflammatory disease that causes joint pain, stiffness and swelling), avascular necrosis (loss of bone caused by insufficient blood supply), traumatic injury (such as a fracture) and bone tumours (which may affect the hip joint).

5.1 Anatomy of the hip

The hip joint is a 'ball and socket joint', which allows for a wide range of movement while at the same time providing a stable joint to facilitate weight-bearing during standing and mobilisation. The joint comprises an articulation between the acetabulum (a 'socket'-shaped area of the pelvis) and the head of the femur (the 'ball'). Stability is provided by a network of ligaments (condensations or thickenings of the joint capsule) that connects the bones of the hip joint. Smooth movement is facilitated by cartilage (a tough substance covering the bone surfaces) and synovial fluid (which provides lubrication to the joint). It is important to be aware that cartilage does not regenerate, so once it has worn away, there is no ability for it to recover.

5.2 Indications for total hip replacement

5.2.1 Osteoarthritis

Osteoarthritis occurs when there is damage to the cartilage in the hip joint, which would usually provide a 'cushion' between the acetabulum and the head of the femur. The cartilage wears and gets progressively thinner until eventually the two bones come into contact. Wear of the bone advances, usually slowly. The process is associated with progressive pain, stiffness and loss of function.

A person generally finds themselves on a waiting list for an elective total hip replacement after months and sometimes years of worsening hip pain, joint stiffness and declining functional ability in both their movement and activities of daily living. Prior to being listed for this surgery, the service user will have trialled alternative management options with their general practitioner and orthopaedic consultant, such as use of mobility aids, medication, joint protection principles, weight loss and exercise. This can be helpful for some people; however, many opt for surgery when these options are no longer providing effective pain relief and/or improved function of the hip. The aim of surgery is to improve independent functioning and pain levels.

5.2.2 Failure of primary total hip replacement

As with any surgical procedure, there are risks of complications following total hip replacement. These include prosthetic wear and loosening, dislocation of the prosthesis and infection to the joint replacement site. These complications can require revision surgery to the joint involving removal of the primary prosthesis and implantation of a new prosthesis. In the case of joint infection, this can be completed as a two-stage procedure whereby the primary prosthesis is removed and an antibiotic-loaded spacer is inserted. Following a period of antibiotic therapy this is then removed and the revision prosthesis implanted.

5.2.3 Fractured neck of femur

Total hip replacement is also carried out following traumatic fracture of the hip (fractured neck of femur). NICE guidance (2011) recommends total hip replacement is offered as the surgical intervention for individuals with a displaced intracapsular fractured neck of femur who:

- were able to walk independently out of doors with no more than the use of a stick and
- are not cognitively impaired and
- are medically fit for anaesthesia and the procedure.

For this cohort of service users, occupational therapy staff should also refer to national hip fracture guidelines (SIGN 2009, NICE 2011) and the quality standard (NICE 2012), together with national falls guidelines (NICE 2013) and professional practice guidelines on the prevention and management of falls (COT 2015a).

5.3 Total hip replacement

A total hip replacement is a surgical procedure that involves the removal of diseased or damaged bone and cartilage in the hip joint, replacing it with an artificial hip joint, known as a prosthesis. This prosthesis is made up of two parts: the 'ball and stem', which is inserted into the femur, and the 'cup socket', which is inserted into the acetabulum. The two parts together make up the new hip, which restores smooth surfaces allowing comfortable movement. Artificial hip joints can be cemented, uncemented or hybrid. A cemented prosthesis is held in place by cement, which attaches the prosthesis to the bone; an uncemented prosthesis has a fine mesh of holes on the surface that the bone grows into; and a hybrid prosthesis has one uncemented component (usually socket), with the other (generally femoral stem) being cemented to the bone. Surgeons will decide with the individual service user which is most suitable.

6 Recommendations and supporting evidence

The recommendation categories reflect areas of importance for service users undergoing total hip replacement and occupational therapy intervention. They are presented in the order of prioritisation identified from the service user consultation (Appendix 3). Where applicable, the qualitative service user feedback has been used to enhance the user perspective as an adjunct to the published evidence.

Recommendations grading

Recommendations are graded from A (high) to D (low) to indicate the **quality** of the evidence.

The scoring of 1 (strong) or 2 (conditional) indicates the **strength** of the recommendation (sections 11.4 and 11.5).

Each statement starts with either '***It is recommended***' or '***It is suggested***'.

'It is recommended . . .' means that most service users would want, or should receive, this course of intervention or action.

'It is suggested . . .' means that the majority of service users would want this intervention but not all, and therefore they should be supported to arrive at a decision for intervention consistent with the benefits and their values and preferences.

Additional details on individual studies (for example, on recruitment numbers and statistically significant p values) can be accessed in the evidence tables (Appendix 7).

This guideline focuses on occupational therapy for adults undergoing total hip replacement, within the context of the multidisciplinary environment. As such, the intervention is specifically occupational therapy, and alternative management options are therefore not explicitly reviewed or discussed. This is in line with the clinical question which indicates that there is no comparator intervention. Benefits and any specific risks are integrally incorporated within the discussion of the evidence.

6.1 Maximised functional independence

Evidence overview – Maximised functional independence
The evidence identified that individual factors, such as co-morbidities and personal history, will affect individual needs and therefore assessments must be individualised and comprehensive. Additionally, the evidence supported taking into account depression, anxiety and cognitive status, as these may have an impact on recovery.

Clear communication by occupational therapists that is consistent with the wider multidisciplinary team can help ensure realistic expectations post-surgery.

To aid with recovery, studies have noted the importance of involving service users in equipment decisions and providing them with advice on pain management.

6.1.1 Introduction

Maximised functional independence focuses on early resumption of activities of daily living (ADLs). It includes assessment and practice with mobility, transfers (from bed, chair, toilet and car), washing and dressing, and domestic activities, such as hot drink preparation. Integral to this is the reinforcement of pre-operative discussions regarding safe movement, incorporating hip precautions as applicable to the individual and in line with local protocols, together with practice in using compensatory equipment. Solutions to specific issues will be discussed on an individual basis.

Although traditionally the domain of the physiotherapist, occupational therapists are increasingly involved in early mobilisation of post-operative service users, including prescription of walking aids. Most service users will be fully weight-bearing, but if partial or no weight-bearing is specified by the surgeon, this must be taught and practised in a functional context.

6.1.2 Evidence

Maximised functional independence

1. ***It is recommended*** that the occupational therapy assessment is comprehensive and considers factors which may affect individual needs, goals, recovery and rehabilitation, including co-morbidities, trauma history, personal circumstances, obesity and pre-operative function. 1C

   (Johansson et al 2010 [C]; Lin and Kaplan 2004 [C]; Marks 2008 [C]; Naylor et al 2008 [C]; Ostendorf et al 2004 [C]; Vincent et al 2007 [C]; Vincent et al 2012 [B]; Wang et al 2010 [C])

   [New evidence 2017]

Limited evidence was identified with respect to occupational therapy and maximising independence in the context of total hip replacement. However, assessment of individual needs underpins occupational therapy practice, and the importance of a comprehensive assessment was highlighted within the evidence.

The literature search identified a strong focus on elective hip replacements, but a number of low-level studies clearly recognised the potential complexities that may be associated with specific individual needs and co-morbidities. While the studies included in this area raised some methodological limitations, they provided evidence of the potential influence of a variety of factors on an individual's needs post-operatively. **Marks (2008)**, for example, retrospectively examined pre-operative functional ability in those with osteoarthritis awaiting a hip replacement, from the perspective of a trauma or non-trauma history. His conclusion was that those who had a history of hip fracture were more functionally impaired prior to surgery and used more assistive devices.

Individual service user characteristics may also impact on functional independence, and additionally length of stay. Body mass index was suggested as being an important consideration when predicting functional outcomes after a hip replacement in the study by **Vincent et al (2007)**. The study concluded that length of stay was significantly greater in the severely obese compared to non-obese, although this contradicts a retrospective cohort study in which body mass index was found to make no difference to length of stay (**Lin and Kaplan 2004**). That study suggested that there was a correlation between increasing age and length of stay, and that co-morbid illnesses were predictive of increased length of stay in the acute rehabilitation setting. **Naylor et al (2008)** identified obesity and/or severe joint disease to be associated with more compromised function, slower mobility and a greater reliance on a walking aid. **Vincent et al (2012)**, in a review of 23 studies on the long-term functional outcomes of hip replacement in obese service users, found that while functional improvement did occur (notably pain reduction and improvement in quality of life), those with obesity did not attain the same level of physical function long-term when compared to non-obese service users.

The variation in these studies, and their individual limitations, means that specific recommendations for occupational therapists have not been made regarding the predictability of functional performance and length of stay in relation to generalised service user characteristics. The main feature of the evidence in this area is to emphasise the vital importance of individualised, person-centred assessment and intervention.

The ability to predict post-operative outcomes, as a means of guiding rehabilitation options, is an area, however, which has been the focus of a number of research studies. In this context, disease-specific outcome measures have featured, with reference to whether their pre-operative scores can facilitate prediction of post-operative outcomes. **Johansson et al (2010)** identified that a poor pre-operative Harris Hip Score was an indicator for poor early post-operative outcomes. Likewise, **Wang et al (2010)** investigated the factors affecting the short-term outcome of primary total hip replacement and developed a multivariate regression equation to predict those short-term outcomes. The Western Ontario and McMaster Universities Osteoarthritis Index (WOMAC) was used and found to be a statistically significant measure that indicated three main factors in predicting total hip replacement outcomes at a minimum of one-year follow-up: pre-operative WOMAC Physical Function Score, gender and pre-operative co-morbidities. Service users with better pre-operative functional scores were likely to have higher post-operative scores, but service users with poorer pre-operative scores were likely to experience greater improvement in function. **Ostendorf et al (2004)**, in a similar vein, set out to define the minimum set of service user reported outcome measures required to assess health status after a total hip replacement, and recommended the use of the Oxford Hip Score and SF-12® health survey in assessment of total hip replacement.

The interest in studies involving disease-specific measures is usefully put in the context of Patient Reported Outcome Measures (PROMs) reported in England (NHS Digital 2017). PROMs for hip replacements have been collected in England since April 2009, aiming to provide information on service users' perceptions of the effectiveness of care delivered in the National Health Service. The Oxford Hip Score is used as the disease-specific measure, and the EQ-5D™ Index and EQ-VAS as a generic measure of self-reported health status. Data reported includes the percentage of respondents reporting joint-related or general health improvements following their operation.

Given that the occupational therapist works as a member of the multidisciplinary team, it is important that while undertaking a comprehensive assessment, the therapist establishes and confirms, but does not duplicate, information that may have already been collected. Where possible, it would be useful for occupational therapists to gain insight into the individual's pre-operative status from any service user reported outcome measures that are being used within their service. It is recognised that access to this information may not always be practicable.

Maximised functional independence	
2. ***It is recommended*** that goal setting is individualised, enhances realistic expectations of functional independence, and commences at pre-operative assessment. *(Hobbs et al 2011 [C]; Judge et al 2011 [C]; Mancuso et al 2003 [C])* [New evidence 2017]	1C
3. ***It is recommended*** that occupational therapists ensure that they provide clear communication and advice that is consistent with that of other members of the multidisciplinary team. *(Drummond et al 2013 [C]; Fielden et al 2003 [C])* [New evidence 2017]	1C

Expectations in relation to surgical outcomes are associated with subsequent post-operative satisfaction. Individual service users will have formed expectations about the likely status of their health and independence following their operation. There is consequently the potential of a mismatch between expectations and likely outcomes, resulting in dissatisfaction post-operatively. Service user expectations were the subject of three large but low-level studies reviewed. A cohort study across 12 European countries (1,108 participants) undertaken by **Hobbs et al (2011)** indicated that service user needs are different from their desires, which in turn may affect satisfaction. It was reported most service user expectations post-surgery related to enabling them to carry out valued activities rather than reversing impairments. **Mancuso et al (2003)** identified in an American study (1,103 participants) that those with worse hip function and overall physical health pre-operatively had greater expectations from the surgery. Decreased functional status pre-operatively was associated with greater importance being placed on post-operative achievement of goals. The most prevalent expectations were in pain relief and improvement in walking.

> *"... after just a couple of months I was walking by myself and able to do just about everything with very little help."*
>
> *Golden Jubilee National Hospital service user feedback (2012)*

In a prospective cohort study in Europe which involved 1,327 participants **(Judge et al 2011)**, a wide variation in service user expectations was identified. Service users with more pre-operative expectations were more likely to have clinically important outcomes 12 months post-total hip replacement.

Fielden et al (2003), in a qualitative study investigating expectations and satisfaction of service users, found that clarity about the roles of the various multidisciplinary team members, and consistent information about post-operative management and discharge planning, were key needs. Although it was a qualitative study, it reinforced the fundamental requirement for effective multidisciplinary working. In the absence of good communication, there is a possibility of conflicting messages or information being received by the service user, which could increase risks and decrease confidence.

Written information is routinely provided to service users, but a descriptive analysis of elective total hip replacement literature provided by occupational therapists in the UK **(Drummond et al 2013)** revealed that literature is inconsistent. This was evident for features such as content, readability and the involvement of service users in their production, with the suggestion that due consideration of the aim, purpose and timing of leaflets is important to ensure that they are fit for purpose.

> *"It is really important that you are given consistent advice from everyone in the team – you can be told different things by different people and this increases your fears and worries both before and after the operation."*
>
> *50+ Forum service user feedback (2012)*
>
> *"Consistency is so important – being given different advice by the nurse, OT, physio and doctor destroys your confidence and trust and faith that they know what they are doing."*
>
> *50+ Forum service user feedback (2012)*

Occupational therapists need to be aware of and discuss the service user's expectations, preferably pre-operatively, as they will influence individual goal setting and satisfaction. Discussion may also include re-directing expectations to a more realistic goal.

Maximised functional independence	
4. ***It is recommended*** that depression and anxiety status are taken into account during pre-operative and post-operative intervention due to their potential for impact on recovery. *(Caracciolo and Giaquinto 2005 [C]; Nickinson et al 2009 [C])*	1C
5. ***It is recommended*** that cognitive status is taken into account during pre-operative and post-operative intervention due to its potential for impact on recovery. *(Wang and Emery 2002 [C]; Wong et al 2002 [C])*	1C

The literature also included studies that considered mental health status, specifically in the context of anxiety and depression. These were low-level, small sample, prospective studies, with the focus being the immediate post-operative period. To determine whether psychological distress and depression were associated with reduced functional improvement following joint replacement, **Caracciolo and Giaquinto (2005)** measured functional recovery and distress. The WOMAC and the Hospital Anxiety and Depression Scale (HAD) measures were administered on admission to a rehabilitation facility (baseline) and then again on discharge (follow-up). The authors found that there was over-threshold depression in their sample of service users following total hip replacement. WOMAC gain scores (function, stiffness and pain) were, however, no different between depressed versus non-depressed service users having total hip replacement. It was suggested that there was therefore no association between psychological distress and depression and functional recovery in this group of service users.

Nickinson et al (2009) investigated the presence and rates of anxiety and depression in post-surgical hip and knee replacement service users. Their findings included that the mean length of stay was five days for depressed or anxious service users compared with four days for non-anxious/depressed service users. On day of discharge, however, the low number of service users whose scores remained above diagnostic level for depression was minimal, suggesting that the depression was a transient phenomenon.

Inpatient occupational therapy intervention is likely to be taking place one to three days post-operatively. It is, therefore, important that the therapist duly considers the service user's potential for depression and anxiety at that time, and that this may impact, albeit temporarily, on motivation or engagement in intervention. Reassurance for the service user and a focus on the fact that in the majority of cases this is a normal experience, rather than an exception, may facilitate recovery.

Cognitive status is also a key individual factor to be identified, and is highlighted within both the NICE and SIGN hip fracture guidelines. The NICE guideline includes a statement that total hip replacement should be offered to those 'not cognitively impaired' (NICE 2011, p11), while the SIGN guideline states that total hip replacement is 'unsuitable for patients with dementia due to the higher dislocation rate' (SIGN 2009, p21).

Wong et al (2002) found that non-confused service users were significantly more independent in performing activities of daily living. While both confused and non-confused groups showed consistent improvement in functional status over time, improvement in the non-confused group was of a greater magnitude. This study had a number of limitations, including the inability to separate out the more detailed analysis in terms of elective compared to fractured neck of femur cases, but emphasised the importance of assessment of cognitive status to assist in identifying complex needs. This is reinforced by the findings of a literature review conducted by **Wang and Emery (2002)**, which, although limited by its lack of review strategy details, highlighted that cognitive impairment affects functional improvement. Of particular note for occupational therapists is that the ability to learn about hip precautions and the use of adaptive behaviours and equipment may be affected by cognitive status.

In the context of cognitive status, while not addressed in the evidence, if occupational therapists are concerned that the service user may lack mental capacity to understand the implications/consent to surgery, they have a professional responsibility to ensure this is brought to the attention of the multidisciplinary team.

The evidence relates to people with dementia; however, consideration should be given to service users with other cognitive difficulties, such as learning disabilities and head injury. It is important to consider a range of reasonable adjustments to ensure that service users with cognitive impairments receive a comprehensive person-centred assessment and are offered appropriate pre- and post-operative treatment. Discussions should include the whole multidisciplinary team, and where applicable carers, to ensure the delivery of safe and effective interventions.

Maximised functional independence	
6. ***It is recommended*** that service users are fully involved in decisions about the equipment required to enable them to carry out daily living activities and to comply with any hip precautions in their home environment post-surgery. *(Thomas et al 2010 [D])*	1D

Assessment and prescription of equipment to facilitate independence and support hip restrictions post-operatively is a key role of the occupational therapist. One of the potential risks associated with equipment is lack of service user compliance, particularly relevant because provision is not just for independence per se but may also be to protect the joint post-surgery (where hip precautions are in use).

Studies examining the provision and use of equipment have been reported in occupational therapy publications, though most of these have been outside of the guideline literature search period. A number of factors are likely to be related to compliance, and an American study by **Thomas et al (2010)** examined the most frequent reasons for non-use of adaptive equipment prescribed by occupational therapists for service users who had returned home following hip replacement surgery. This small study involved telephone interviews with ten service users, 78% of whom reported they had little or no inclusion in the decision making about equipment. While a very low-level study, which may have some lack of generalisation to the UK given that respondents in the study had to purchase equipment, it provided support for a recommendation that decisions around equipment requirements must involve the service user. The influence of the individual's home environment on non-use of equipment was also highlighted, mentioning examples such as issues of convenience for others and existing home design features.

It is important to note, however, that equipment provision in the UK is not universally free, and the types of equipment prescribed or available are variable. The need to purchase equipment can add another dimension and further highlights the importance of service user involvement in decisions. A strong focus on education and the purpose of the equipment and risks associated with non-compliance may be important to inspire use.

Maximised functional independence	
7. ***It is recommended*** that service users are given advice on effective pain management strategies, to decrease pre-operative pain experience and sleep disturbance, and enhance post-operative physical function. *(Berge et al 2004 [B]; Montin et al 2007 [C]; Parsons et al 2009 [C])*	1B

A potential influence on function is the experience of pain. **Berge et al (2004)** implemented a small, randomised controlled trial, rated as a moderate level of evidence, in which a core aim was to investigate the effects and impact of a pre-operative pain management programme on pain. Information on blinding and co-morbidities was lacking and therefore the study had some methodological weaknesses. Assessment included use of the Arthritis Impact Scale (AIMS) pre- and post-operatively, one finding being that at one-year follow-up, the treatment group had statistically significant better scores for the AIMS physical activity score. This study also identified that pain management advice could decrease average pain intensity, distress and pain-related sleep disturbance. The importance of pain management was reflected in another study **(Montin et al 2007)**, in which pre-operative pain was found to have an association, though not statistically significant, with increased anxiety and reduced health-related quality of life post-surgery. The impact of uncontrolled pain on mood was also highlighted in a qualitative study exploring the lived experiences of service users with severe osteoarthritis awaiting joint surgery **(Parsons et al 2009)**.

Pain management has a number of facets and is an area of intervention which may be addressed by one or more members of the multidisciplinary team. Occupational therapists may not always contribute specifically to this intervention at pre-operative assessment, but their role in this area, particularly in relation to joint protection and energy conservation management, should be recognised. Additionally, this is relevant when considering post-operative rehabilitation, to maximise function and effective pain management. While evidence on the occupational therapist's role in pain management was not specifically targeted in this guideline's literature search strategy, it is an area of practice where occupational therapists can contribute to the multidisciplinary intervention.

Maximised functional independence

8. ***It is suggested*** that standardised assessment and outcome measures are used, where appropriate, to determine functional outcomes and occupational performance in rehabilitation settings, either inpatient or community based. 2C

   (Alviar et al 2011 [B]; Gillen et al 2007 [C]; Kiefer and Emery 2004 [C]; Oberg et al 2005 [D])

[New evidence 2017]

Evidence on the use of occupational therapy standardised assessments or outcome measures as part of intervention with service users receiving a total hip replacement was lacking in the literature identified. Three small-scale and low-level evidence primary research studies were appraised which focused on functional performance. The newer review, while moderate quality evidence, reported from a different perspective and hence the overall grade of the evidence was not uplifted (see section 11.5).

The Canadian Occupational Performance Measure (COPM©) was used in one study to rate service user functional abilities in activities of daily living, specifically focusing on community activities **(Gillen et al 2007)**. The ratings were self-reported performance and satisfaction with performance. The study identified that COPM© provides a valid and reliable method to evaluate community functioning based on self-report.

COPM© was also used as an outcome measure pre-operatively and at follow-up after total hip replacement in a Swedish study **(Oberg et al 2005)**. Findings indicated a reduction in the number and severity of problems and a statistically significant improvement in both performance and satisfaction using this measure. This study also used the Functional Assessment System (FAS) of lower extremity dysfunction and the generic health survey SF-36®. In the SF-36® data, service users showed a statistically significant improvement in almost all domains, and the FAS showed statistically significant improvements in the variables reflecting lower extremity functions related to hip problems. The authors suggested that all the instruments delivered important information on the functional and activity status of service users.

In the third study, **Kiefer and Emery (2004)** used the Functional Independence Measure (FIM™) to look at the functional gains in self-care, mobility and locomotion of service users, and found that it was able to identify improvement in functional performance.

A review was undertaken by **Alviar et al (2011)** of eight patient-reported outcome measures in which the measure concepts were linked to the International Classification of Functioning, Disability and Health. Whilst activity and participation concepts had the most representation (61%), environmental factors were not addressed in the majority of tools, indicating the need for caution in the selection of a tool to demonstrate therapy outcomes.

The value of standardised assessments and outcome measures in the acute setting is fully recognised. However, expert opinion from the guideline development group is that the use of these routinely can be challenging, particularly given the short length of stay and limited opportunity for therapist intervention during elective inpatient care. It is also relevant to note that given the core treatment is the total hip replacement surgery, and that intervention involves a multidisciplinary approach, it can be difficult to extract the occupational therapy-specific contribution to the service user's outcomes, particularly in the short time span.

Service users requiring further intervention or rehabilitation, potentially more likely following a traumatic history to the hip replacement or complex individual needs, may receive this either in the community or as an inpatient. In these situations the use of standardised assessment and outcome measures is recommended and should be incorporated as part of specific goal-orientated intervention. The evidence identified from the literature search was not sufficient, however, to recommend a specific standardised assessment or outcome measure. Occupational therapists should, therefore, additionally review the general evidence available when making their decision about the most appropriate tools for their practice.

6.2 Reduced anxiety

Evidence overview – Reduced anxiety
The evidence highlights the anxiety service users may have about their hip operation and points to a number of practices that may help to reduce this, such as the pre-operative provision of equipment. For most service users, pre-operative education given in a clinic setting is appropriate, but individual context needs to be considered. Studies also investigated the type and presentation of information that could be considered best practice. While these may be a useful reference point, they will need to be balanced against any occupational therapy service constraints.

6.2.1 Introduction

Hip replacement surgery is seen as an 'extensive life event', consisting of a number of phases for the individual. **Gustafsson et al (2010)** explored the meaning of hip surgery to five individuals, a study which emphasised the issues involved with making the decision for surgery. The author identified a core theme from respondents of 'choosing the challenge', with highlighted sub-themes of getting ready for the operation and the associated hopes and fears. This 'life event' is for many service users accompanied by anxiety.

> *"This is a common and routine operation so sometimes you feel all the pre-operative assessment is a 'tick box' – but to you it is a major event and very worrying."*
>
> *50+ Forum service user feedback (2012)*

Pre-operative assessment and intervention can be an opportune time to explore those anxieties which the service user may be experiencing. Occupational therapists are frequently involved pre-operatively and it is important at this point to distinguish between pre-operative individualised assessment and pre-operative education. Individualised assessment should involve a one-to-one assessment, while education may be delivered on an individual or group basis by one or more members of the multidisciplinary team and follow a more prescribed programme. Both formats should allow the opportunity for the service user to express concerns and/or ask questions.

6.2.2 Evidence

Reduced anxiety	
9. ***It is recommended*** that the pre-operative assessment undertaken by the occupational therapist allows adequate time for individualised questions and discussion of expectations and anxieties. *(Fielden et al 2003 [C]; McDonald et al 2014 [A]; McDonald et al 2004 [A]; Montin et al 2007 [C])* [New evidence 2017]	1A
10. ***It is suggested*** that occupational therapists offer support and advice to service users who may be anxious about an accelerated discharge home. *(Heine et al 2004 [D]; Hunt et al 2009 [D]; Montin et al 2007 [C])*	2C

A number of sources of evidence were identified relating to anxiety that may be experienced by a service user during the various stages of the pathway for hip replacement surgery.

A Cochrane review **(McDonald et al 2004)** suggested that there was insufficient evidence to support or refute the use of pre-operative education to improve post-operative outcomes, especially in terms of functioning and length of stay. There was the suggestion, however, that pre-operative education may have beneficial effects when targeted to reduce anxiety and for those most in need of support, for example those with greater disability and/or limited social support. There was overall evidence that pre-operative education had a modest beneficial effect on pre-operative anxiety. In the subsequent updated review **(McDonald et al 2014)**, the findings again indicated that there was lack of certainty about the benefits, over and above usual care, in relation to reducing anxiety, surgical outcomes (for example pain and function) and adverse events. Whilst the quality of evidence was low, the potential for some benefit when pre-education is considered in the context of an individual's physical, psychological and social needs was highlighted in the 2014 review, with particular reference to those with depression, anxiety or unrealistic expectations.

The importance of an individually tailored approach to the pre-operative assessment was also highlighted in the evidence. **Montin et al (2007)** found those who were older and overweight experienced greater anxiety before surgery. Given that these individuals and others with co-morbidities may have slower recovery, this study reinforced the important role of effective and individualised pre-operative assessment. The importance of time to ask questions of an individual nature was also raised in the qualitative study by **Fielden et al (2003)**, where service users identified that there was a lack of scheduled time for them to ask questions pre- or post-operatively.

> *"I would like to take this opportunity to thank all staff for their excellent help and assistance with answers to all my questions.*
>
> *"I was well advised, supported and made ready to go home early. I was well prepared pre-operatively."*
>
> *Golden Jubilee National Hospital service user feedback (2012)*

In another study, service users with accelerated discharge described concerns and anxieties about the consequences of early discharge for them or their family, especially regarding managing pain, mobility at home and support needs **(Hunt et al 2009)**. **Heine et al (2004)** in a small qualitative study similarly identified that service users needed to feel safe and secure about their return home, and that this can be enhanced by providing information at a pre-operative stage as well as prior to discharge.

Occupational therapists may not always have the opportunity to discuss concerns post-operatively in detail due to the limited time that the service user is on the ward. It is important, wherever possible, to ensure these issues are addressed during pre-operative assessment.

Reduced anxiety	
11. ***It is recommended*** that pre-operative assessment and education is carried out in the most appropriate environment for the service user. For the majority of service users a clinic environment is appropriate, but where needs are complex, a home assessment should be an available option. *(Crowe and Henderson 2003 [B]; Drummond et al 2012 [C]; Orpen and Harris 2010 [C]; Rivard et al 2003 [B])*	1B
12. ***It is suggested*** that provision of equipment pre-operatively may facilitate familiarity and confidence in use. *(Fielden et al 2003 [C]; Orpen and Harris 2010 [C])*	2C
13. ***It is suggested*** that service users may value being treated by the same occupational therapist throughout the process, from pre-operative assessment/education to post-operative rehabilitation wherever possible. *(Spalding 2003 [C])*	2C
14. ***It is suggested*** that occupational therapists should contribute to standardised pre-operative education interventions, providing information, advice and demonstrations where relevant (e.g. of joint protection principles, equipment). *(Coudeyre et al 2007 [B]; Johansson et al 2007 [B]; Spalding 2003 [C]; Spalding 2004 [C]; Soever et al 2010 [C])*	2B

The setting for pre-operative intervention could potentially be in the clinic or within the individual's home.

The benefits of pre-operative home-based occupational therapy intervention were explored from the perspective of ten service users in a small qualitative study **(Orpen and Harris 2010)**. Pre-operative occupational therapy intervention consisted of performance of activities of daily living, environmental considerations and social considerations. The analysis resulted in the identification of five main themes:

- Pre-operative equipment use increased independence, progress and confidence. The belief that installation of equipment pre-operatively would have relieved anxiety and provided the opportunity to try out equipment was also identified as a potential need in the qualitative work of **Fielden et al (2003)**.
- Individual needs are better met through timely visits.
- Home intervention by a competent therapist offered reassurance regarding surgery.
- Knowing one's home environment is suitable increased confidence in planning hospital discharge after surgery.
- Establishing the social support networks available on discharge was important in pre-operative assessment and planning.

A key study limitation was the potential for recall bias given that the timing of the interviews ranged from five weeks to six months post-surgery; however, it provided useful information about what is important to service users prior to hip replacement.

A Canadian study, with well-controlled confounding variables, provided more robust evidence. **Rivard et al (2003)** in their case control study examined the location and nature of pre-operative occupational therapy assessment/intervention. One group received a pre-operative home visit one to two weeks prior to surgery together with one-to-one teaching in their own home when the therapists were able to assess the home environment directly. The other group attended a pre-operative assessment clinic at the hospital, also within one to two weeks of their surgery, and received their teaching in a group setting, with therapists relying on service user/family reports for information about the home environment. The outcomes of this study indicated that the allocation of resources to one-to-one pre-operative home visits cannot be supported, given that similar intervention can be carried out in a facility-based setting requiring far fewer resources (staff time, travel costs) and achieving the same outcomes; that is, there was no significant difference between length of stay and discharge destination.

In a second Canadian study, a randomised controlled trial similarly investigated pre-operative interventions **(Crowe and Henderson 2003)**. The control group received one standard pre-operative clinic visit one to two weeks prior to surgery, which included any medical tests and other assessments. The service user was briefly educated about what to bring to hospital, instructions about pre-operative preparation, information about the hospital stay and immediate post-operative phase (including functional implications of surgery and temporary post-operative functional limitations). The intervention group received individually tailored multidisciplinary rehabilitation to optimise functional capacity, education about the in-hospital phase and early discharge planning. The occupational therapy component comprised environmental preparation, education, strategies to improve pre-operative functioning, energy consideration and task simplification. Some received a home visit to plan environmental changes. All service users in the rehabilitation intervention group received interdisciplinary counselling/education focused on preparation for discharge home.

The study found that a pre-operative, individually tailored rehabilitation programme reduced length of hospital stay, and that service users were less anxious before surgery and were better prepared in advance for their return home. The length of stay result contradicts that found in other studies, but the impact of pre-operative intervention on reducing anxiety is reinforced. While this study is a valuable piece of evidence, there were variations between the groups and the completeness of data, and not all participants received a re-assessment of their anxiety.

Coudeyre et al (2007) reviewed the literature to assist in the development of guidelines for pre-operative rehabilitation for hip and knee total replacement in France. In summarising the findings, Coudeyre et al indicated the importance of individualised intervention and advocated that *'pre-operative multidisciplinary rehabilitation, comprising at least occupational therapy and education is desirable among the most fragile patients'* (Coudeyre et al 2007, p195).

"The home visit by my local OT was extremely helpful. He explained very clearly what I might expect and ways of helping my recovery and improving my post-op mobility."

Golden Jubilee National Hospital service user feedback (2012)

"Home visits are the single most important factor – you feel in control when the OT comes to your home and more able to talk through any worries. A home visit as part of the pre-operative assessment for those who live alone is really important."

50+ Forum service user feedback (2012)

The framework for provision of pre-operative intervention by the occupational therapist will have geographical variations. The opportunity to provide a home visit, which may be the preferred option, may not always be feasible due to limitations of resources (staff, time available) if the service user lives outside the catchment area of the hospital or is treated as part of a regional/national programme. A national survey of occupational therapy practice in the UK identified that home visits were not routinely carried out by occupational therapists, either pre-operatively or post-operatively **(Drummond et al 2012)**. Home visits were 'sporadic' and usually associated with specific service user needs such as co-morbidities, living alone, frailty, a history of falls or having no one to measure furniture heights. The nature of service provision and resources may also provide a barrier to the provision of equipment pre-operatively, influenced particularly by local community equipment service arrangements.

In summary, the evidence indicates that pre-operative occupational therapy intervention can be provided effectively via the clinic setting for most individuals. Where the service user has complex needs, then home-based provision should be an option to optimise pre-surgery function and enhance the rehabilitation and discharge planning process.

Given the volume of total hip replacements undertaken, routine home-based intervention would potentially be resource intensive and, therefore, prohibitively high cost. While not perhaps explicit within the evidence, it is, therefore, important that where needs are complex, the occupational therapist makes contact with any community services/agencies or family carers involved. This can facilitate the gathering of information, which may inform decision making with respect to the need for a home assessment and determine the potential support available to advise/prepare the service user pre-admission. It is considered essential by the guideline development group that there is the option of a home assessment in the management of complex individual needs.

Spalding conducted qualitative work with service users who had experienced occupational therapy in pre-admission education sessions **(Spalding 2004)**. The study investigated the perspectives of ten service users and seven health professionals involved in a pre-education programme consisting of a two-hour session. The session included explanation, demonstration and opportunity for service user participation and questions. The beneficial outcome of service user empowerment was explored, identifying themes of confidence, trust, control, responsibility, involvement, knowledge, support and understanding.

An earlier article by Spalding reporting on the same study focused on pre-operative education and anxiety **(Spalding 2003)**, and found that service user education can reduce anxiety. This was achieved by enabling service users to understand the experiences that will be encountered during and after surgery; that is, the chronological experience of total hip replacement. Spalding also identified that demonstrations were easier to understand and facilitated learning, and that making the unknown familiar through an opportunity to meet staff who would be involved in care on the ward was valued by respondents.

While it is preferable that the occupational therapist who assesses the service user/ provides education is the therapist who provides the intervention post-operatively, this may not always be feasible. This may be affected by pre-operative and surgery time scales and factors such as rotational staff or staff leave.

A randomised controlled trial in Finland **(Johansson et al 2007)** set out to determine whether it was possible to increase service user knowledge and certainty about care-related issues, to reach a more empowering learning experience, and to exercise a more positive impact on selected clinical outcomes by additional pre-admission education. One group received standard written education and non-systematic oral education while the intervention group received face-to-face education with nurses trained in the concept map method, plus the written educational material. Pre-admission education using the concept map method and written education was found to yield better learning results than the use of written education material with non-systematic oral education. However, it was also suggested that written information is more effective than verbal, so services should therefore be employing both strategies for pre-admission education.

Soever et al (2010) aimed to identify the educational needs of adults having hip or knee replacement surgery through a small qualitative study. This revealed that the topics of interest to service users included knowing the team, condition information and management, waiting list priorities, pre-operative activities, preparing for admission, the rehabilitation process, functional recovery and follow-up. They also identified factors affecting educational needs (why education is important); that is, fears, family information needs and expectations. Soever et al concluded by suggesting the use of a comprehensive checklist for an education programme, the content of which may be a useful reference point for occupational therapists.

While it is beneficial to provide information in a variety of formats to meet, for example, learning style preferences, literacy and language skills or sensory needs, this may not always be feasible depending on the resources available to a team.

6.3 Resumption of meaningful occupation

Evidence overview – Resumption of meaningful occupation

The evidence shows that post-operative expectations often focus first on physical recovery, and as that progresses, the resumption of roles becomes important. However, resumption of these roles can be impeded by lack of confidence and unrealistic expectations.

As hip replacements are increasingly occurring in younger age groups, return to work can be a key goal of some service users. The evidence underlines that this can be a realistic goal for many, with studies showing most service users who want to return to work do, though the demands of the job and individual circumstances play a part. Another goal may be the return to sports or physical activities, although the evidence points to a very limited increase in physical activities post-operatively. Occupational therapists can help service users overcome barriers to resuming these types of roles.

6.3.1 Introduction

Occupational roles, whether these be employment, housework or caring for others, are important to individual wellbeing. After the acute hospital phase has been completed, some service users may require support in order to facilitate resumption of activities required for those occupational roles. The continuation of therapy input, particularly relating to work and leisure needs, may be more appropriately addressed in the community.

Intervention and support in the community may be delivered by a variety of service providers, including health (hospital or community based), social services and private providers. These community services may take the form of outpatient teams, intermediate care teams, reablement/enablement teams or outreach teams. Community services may be provided within the home setting or in clinics or outpatient centres. Seamless service provision is important to enable wider goals set by the service user at initial assessment to be continued as their journey progresses from the inpatient episode through to continued rehabilitation in the community, addressing any issues the person may encounter during their daily routine.

Facilitating longer-term reintegration into community activities is not an area where occupational therapy intervention is routinely implemented following an elective hip replacement. This is more likely following a hip fracture, or when there are complex needs following elective surgery. It is important, however, that the service user is encouraged to consider activities they wish to engage in subsequent to the immediate post-operative period, and to discuss how they may re-engage in past occupations or become involved in new physical or social activities.

Post-operative rehabilitation to facilitate community reintegration is frequently and most likely to be provided via reablement, community services and day hospitals. However, resources may not always exist, which may cause a barrier to provision. Further rehabilitation may, therefore, need to be promoted by encouraging the service user and their family to be proactive in facilitating self-rehabilitation.

Inability to work can have a significant impact on an individual and their family and may be a key occupational role that a service user wishes to return to. The average age for total hip replacement from the various data sources in the UK is 67–69 years, yet while many service users receiving a hip replacement are retired, there are increasing numbers of younger individuals receiving surgery due to improved prosthesis life. Additionally, with the fact that in the future the retirement age will potentially be later, and that individuals may be involved in voluntary or other work-related activities, work roles are an area which should not be neglected.

> *"This [work roles] must be considered in the widest sense – some people are no longer in paid work but do voluntary work which is really important to them."*
>
> *50+ Forum service user feedback (2012)*

Ideally, work-related issues should be addressed earlier in the care pathway of arthritis to facilitate adaptation to the work environment while the individual is still at work and not yet listed for surgery.

It is important that occupational therapists, where necessary, access guidance and information on work-related assessment and intervention, such as the *Work matters* resources available from their professional body, the Royal College of Occupational Therapists (COT and National Social Inclusion Programme 2007).

6.3.2 Evidence

Resumption of meaningful occupation	
15. ***It is recommended*** that work roles are discussed at the earliest opportunity as part of a comprehensive assessment. *(Bohm 2010 [C]; Cowie et al 2013 [C]; Malviya et al 2014 [A]; Mobasheri et al 2006 [D]; Nunley et al 2011 [C]; Sankar et al 2013 [C])* [New evidence 2017]	1C
16. ***It is suggested*** that for service users who are working, advice is provided relating to maintaining their work role pre-operatively, post-operative expectations and relevant information for employers. *(Bohm 2010 [C]; Cowie et al 2013 [C]; Malviya et al 2014 [A]; Mobasheri et al 2006 [D]; Nunley et al 2011 [C]; Parsons et al 2009 [D]; Sankar et al 2013 [C])* [New evidence 2017]	2C

A systematic review and six studies providing low-level evidence were identified with a focus on the relationship between work and total hip replacement.

Cowie et al (2013) undertook a study in the UK involving 239 participants under the age of 65 years, finding a mean length of time of 13.9 weeks for return to work, and return without restrictions for 78% of participants. It was identified that activities at work may be limited initially and return may take longer for those with a high body mass index. **Sankar et al (2013)** similarly found that more than half of the 166 individuals, whose mean age was mid-50s, had returned to work by three months post-surgery, with the majority experiencing fewer limitations than pre-surgery.

A systematic review undertaken by **Malviya et al (2014)** investigated the evidence for those factors which influenced employment outcomes following total hip replacement. Factors of importance were age, motivation, employment before surgery and the nature of the job. Those who were younger with fewer co-morbidities were more likely to return to work; and where heavy manual labour was involved, return was slower. The importance of exploring expectations in relation to return to work was highlighted, given that unrealistic expectations could lead to poorer recovery. It was also identified that those unemployed, off sick for longer pre-operatively or on benefits were less likely to obtain or return to work.

Nunley et al (2011) explored the area of return to work for younger service users in America through a multi-centre telephone study. The study found that most young active individuals who were employed before their surgery could be expected to return to work (90.4%) and the vast majority returned to their pre-operative occupation. This was similar to results in the smaller retrospective study by **Mobasheri et al (2006)**, who likewise found that nearly all service users who were working pre-operatively returned to their jobs. Nunley's cohort enabled analysis of 790 responses, but specifically targeted younger adults, with a mean age at time of surgery of 49.5 years, considerably younger than the typical adult receiving a total hip replacement in the UK. Older respondents (although upper age limit in the study was 65 for men and 55 for women) were found to report more restrictions at work and difficulties with particular activities such as squatting, kneeling, driving and climbing. **Bohm (2010)** in a small cohort study also found that total hip replacement had a positive effect on work capacity for those service users who returned to work.

A further qualitative study by **Parsons et al (2009)** explored the experiences of service users living with severe osteoarthritis while awaiting hip and knee joint replacement surgery and highlighted the difficulty of maintaining work or the need to seek premature retirement. The study also made reference to a lack of understanding on the part of the employer.

These studies reinforce that closer attention may need to be given to service users who are still in the workforce in terms of discussing their job roles and supporting return to work. In the context of the wider clinical pathway, this could mean occupational therapists providing advice on areas such as energy conservation, joint protection, pacing and possible role/task modification while awaiting hip replacement. Discussion around employment status should form part of the pre-operative assessment, to give the service user a realistic time frame regarding return to work and allowing them to plan a return to work schedule with their employer. Post-operatively, this should also be addressed, with advice given regarding when the service user can return to completing certain tasks as opposed to others, and giving suggestions about task and environmental adaptations to promote a successful transition back to work post-operatively. Where resources are available it may be appropriate to refer on to community services for return to work programme intervention.

Acute hospital staff may not always have the opportunity to gain experience in managing issues or questions related to employment. An added concern may be that a service user's expectations may be raised and then cannot be followed up. The potential lack of community resources to which service users can be referred, where further support or advice is needed in relation to work, may be an additional barrier.

Resumption of meaningful occupation

17. ***It is recommended*** that occupational therapists provide advice to facilitate service users to establish previous and new roles and relationships, and shift their focus from disability to ability. 1C

(Grant et al 2009 [C]; McHugh and Luker 2012 [C])

[New evidence 2017]

A more general focus on resumption of roles and relationships following a total hip replacement was identified as a key theme in a small qualitative study, which investigated the processes of recovery from the service user perspective **(Grant et al 2009)**. The study highlighted that the physical domain was seen as being the main focus of recovery in hospital, but as recovery progressed, psychosocial issues, such as re-establishing roles and relationships, and shifting the focus from pre-surgical disability to post-operative ability, could be challenging. However, reliance on others for assistance with everyday activities decreased and this facilitated the re-establishment of roles and relationships and the expansion of horizons.

Grant et al explored the re-establishment of relationships, although the focus reported was on activities such as going out, gardening and visiting friends. Sexual activity within relationships was not apparently raised by participants, although this is an area which can be an important aspect of resumption of roles. Service users should be given the opportunity to discuss this issue, although it is suggested this is most likely to be within the context of protocols to avoid the risk of dislocation. A national survey of occupational therapy practice **(Drummond et al 2012)** identified that the discussion of sexual activities was reported by only 5 out of the 174 respondents within the 'other ADL' category.

In a qualitative study, **McHugh and Luker (2012)** interviewed 25 individuals in the UK six months after a total hip replacement regarding whether their expectations had been met. Disappointment in time for recovery was a feature of participant responses, with the expression of uncertainty about whether their progress was going 'well', and a feeling of being disabled. Building confidence and receiving feedback were identified as two of the challenges of recovery, despite successful joint replacement.

The focus on early discharge may mean that the issues arising in terms of resuming previous roles and taking on new ones may not always be apparent or possible to address during the acute hospital phase.

Resumption of meaningful occupation	
18. ***It is recommended*** that occupational therapists encourage early discussion and goal setting for community reintegration. *(de Groot et al 2008 [D]; Gillen et al 2007 [C]; Heiberg et al 2013 [D]; McHugh and Luker 2012 [C]; Smith et al 2015 [B])* [Statement amended, new evidence 2017	1C
19. ***It is suggested*** that the return to physical and sporting activities is considered within an occupational therapy assessment and interventions. *(Abe et al 2014 [C]; Cowie et al 2013 [C]; Harding et al 2014 [C]; Ollivier et al 2014 [C]; Vissers et al 2013 [C]; Wagenmakers et al 2011 [C]; Williams et al 2012 [C]; Wilson and Villar 2011 [D])* [New statement and evidence 2017]	2C
20. ***It is suggested*** that where specific needs are identified, the occupational therapist refers the service user on to community rehabilitation, reablement or intermediate care services to enhance community reintegration. *(de Groot et al 2008 [D]; Gillen et al 2007 [C])*	2C

A systematic review **(Smith et al 2015)** assessed the evidence on attitudes, perceptions and expectations of physical activity post-total hip replacement. Expectations compared to pre-joint disease levels were low with regard to participating in greater sports or physical activities and, where desired, often inhibited by limitations or inconsistency in advice or education. The authors suggest that there is a need to develop confidence and facilitate greater levels of physical activity. This could be achieved through education on the likely progression of physical activity following surgery, together with ensuring that targets for physical activity and social integration are individualised.

McHugh and Luker's (2012) study, as described earlier, also identified the issue of diminished confidence, especially in the context of participants' hopes that there would have been a substantial improvement in mobility and, as such, return to leisure pursuits and hobbies at an earlier time. The authors identify the importance of discussion of expectations to avoid 'false optimism'. Desired functional improvements were the subject of the qualitative research undertaken by **Heiberg et al (2013)** in which the views of 64 Norwegian participants were sought before the total hip replacement, and at 3 and 12 months post-surgery. Personal care tasks were identified as the key focus at 3 months, with attention returning by 12 months to the pre-operative aspirations related to recreation, leisure and mobility and moving around activities. Both these studies, and the **Smith et al (2015)** review, highlight the need to consider the longer-term return to activities, as well as the more immediate post-operative goals.

Sporting activity may range from low impact (e.g. static cycling, golf, walking and swimming) to high impact (e.g. football, contact sports and jogging). The return to physical and sporting activities post-total hip replacement is the subject of a growing body of research, particularly given the demand and advances in joint replacement and availability of hip replacement to those of a younger age (**Wilson and Villar 2011**). A total hip replacement, with its impact on reducing pain and increasing physical function, could be predicted to result in an increase in physical activity post-operatively.

The impact of total hip replacement on physical activity levels was examined in an American study carried out by **Harding et al (2014)**. Data was obtained pre-operatively, using an accelerometer, from 19 individuals awaiting a total hip replacement, and subsequently at six months post-operatively. The findings indicated that there was no change in the physical activity or its intensity over time following the joint replacement; at six months, 83% of time was spent in sedentary activities, compared to 82% pre-operatively. **Wagenmakers et al (2011)** also investigated self-reported physical activity behaviour of 653 participants at one year post-total hip replacement. The prospective Dutch multicentre cohort study identified that most time was spent in household and leisure activities, with age (over 75 years) and higher body mass index being important determinants with respect to lower levels of activity. **Williams et al (2012),** in an American retrospective study, also found younger age and lower body mass index to be key variables in predicting a University of California, Los Angeles (UCLA) activity score of seven or more at one year, with gender (male) and pre-operative activity being two other important variables.

An earlier cohort study in the Netherlands **(de Groot et al 2008)** identified that actual physical activity on objective measurement had not increased as much as expected at six months following hip surgery (0.7% improvement compared to baseline measures). The activity measured with an activity monitor included movement-related activities (for example, walking and cycling) together with body postures (sitting and standing) and changes in body posture (for example, sit to stand movements). Service users self-reported the time spent in recreational, household and occupational activities, using a modification of the Physical Activity Scale for the Elderly. There was, however, variation between the objectively measured activity data and service user self-reported accounts. Service users reported an 86% increase in activity. The outcomes were measured six months post-operatively, a relatively short period of time following major surgery, and there may have been some self-report bias. The de Groot et al research team undertook a subsequent study to examine the recovery of different aspects of physical functioning at a period of nearly four years post-total hip replacement **(Vissers et al 2013)**. Twenty-three of the original total hip replacement cohort participated, with the findings indicating that daily activity level was lower than at the six-month timeline, although there were, as before, perceived ongoing improvements in physical function capacity and performance of activities of daily living.

Given the potentially low level of physical and daily living activity, even within a relatively healthy study population, it is considered important that service users' needs and goals for 'activity' be identified.

Abe et al (2014) focused specifically on jogging as a physical activity in research involving 527 participants who had received a total hip replacement and 81 in receipt of hip resurfacing arthroplasty (mean age 62 years). In this Japanese study, post-operative jogging was undertaken by 13 total hip replacement participants (a further 10 who jogged had received hip resurfacing arthroplasty); a total of 33 individuals across the study had habitually jogged pre-operatively. Those participants who indicated an interest in jogging, but were not participating in the activity, identified reasons which included: anxiety, physical status (such as pain, decreased range of movement and muscle weakness) and lumbar or knee pain. Post-surgery follow-up (mean 4.8 years) identified no reports of pain or evidence from radiographs of hip loosening.

Ollivier et al (2014) investigated participation in sport after total hip replacement in a French study, with 366 of 571 participants followed up (mean period of 9.8 years) indicating they had resumed sporting activity. Fear of dislocation, avoiding wear and surgeon recommendations were the main reasons for not engaging in sport, with factors such as pre-operative function, motivation, duration of symptoms and post-operative satisfaction correlating with the level of participation. The mean time between the surgery and the return to sporting activity was reported as 6.6 months. The study undertaken by **Cowie et al (2013)** likewise considered return to sporting activities. Those with a lower body mass index returned to sporting activities earlier, with resumption of sports or similar physical activities taking place at a mean of 18.8 weeks.

A study carried out in America **(Gillen et al 2007)** examined the effect of occupational therapy intervention that focused on improving community skills post-operatively. Activities targeted were based on five pre-determined goals, specifically entering and exiting a vehicle, shopping, managing outdoor obstacles, participating safely in the community and travelling to and from outpatient appointments. The intervention took place in a single 45-minute session and the study involved 107 individuals who had received either a hip or knee replacement. Performance and satisfaction with performance were measured using an adapted version of the Canadian Occupational Performance Measure. Confidence was measured with a researcher-designed scale.

Outcomes were positive, with overall higher ratings on all measures post-intervention, indicating the benefit of practice within the natural environment. It should be noted that the occupational therapy intervention was provided via a private rehabilitation centre, the measures were self-reported and there was no follow-up to determine the longer-term benefits. To optimise rehabilitation outcomes, there should be a focus on enhancing community participation and decreasing activity limitations.

The focus of acute intervention is likely to mean a strong concentration on fitness for discharge. It is, however, important that the pre-operative assessment in particular provides advice and suggestions for goals that the service user can work towards once they have returned home. The acute sector occupational therapy service is unlikely to have the resources available to provide the kind of follow-up community intervention as described by Gillen et al (2007), and therefore onward referral is most likely to be indicated. The potential of reablement/rehabilitation services post-total hip replacement may be significantly impacted by the availability of local services and the eligibility criteria. Encouraging and empowering the service user with tools and confidence to be pro-active in achieving long-term goals without therapist input is therefore important.

6.4 Hip precautions

Evidence overview – Hip precautions

The evidence is largely inconclusive on the benefits of implementing hip precautions or the risks of removing hip precautions. Many studies showed improved service user satisfaction, earlier functional independence and no higher risk of dislocation after the removal of hip precautions, but these studies did have considerable limitations. From a practitioner perspective, the evidence points to variation in practice when it comes to advising service users on hip precautions, with practitioners identifying a need for more high-quality research on the impact of relaxing or removing precautions on dislocations and rehabilitation outcomes.

6.4.1 Introduction

Dislocation is one of the potential complications of total hip replacement. A total of 8,367 hip revision procedures was reported in England and Wales in 2015, the most frequent procedure being a single-stage revision (86%). Dislocation accounted for 15% of single-stage revisions, with aseptic loosening 51% and infection 3% (National Joint Registry 2016, pp76–77). A large multi-surgeon audit carried out in 2008 reported 3.4% of service users undergoing primary total hip replacement experienced dislocation (Blom et al 2008). Of the single episodes of dislocation reported in that study, 77.3% occurred within three months of surgery, highlighting that dislocation is more likely in the three months post-operatively.

Variations in practice exist, but to avoid the risk of dislocation, 'hip precaution' protocols have commonly been put in place. An inconsistency in approach to hip precautions was highlighted in particular by occupational therapists as part of the guideline topic identification process. The potential, therefore, for the development of practice guideline recommendations for occupational therapists in this area has been seen as desirable and, as such, remained a hot topic at the time of the guideline review.

6.4.2 Evidence

Hip precautions	
21. ***It is recommended*** that occupational therapists consult with the surgical team regarding any specific precautions to be followed post-operatively. *(Barnsley et al 2015 [B]; Hol et al 2010 [B]; McQuaid et al 2014 [C]; Peak et al 2005 [B]; Restrepo et al 2011 [B]; Smith et al 2016 [A]; Stewart and McMillan 2011 [C]; van der Weegen et al 2016 [B]; Ververeli et al 2009 [B])* [New evidence 2017]	1B
22. ***It is recommended*** that occupational therapists advise service users, where protocol includes precautions, on appropriate position behaviours for those daily activities applicable to the individual's needs, ranging from getting in/out of a car to answering the telephone. *(Coole et al 2013 [C]; Drummond et al 2012 [C]; Malik et al 2002 [D]; Peak et al 2005 [B]; Smith and Sackley 2016 [C]; Stewart and McMillan 2011 [C]; Ververeli et al 2009 [B])* [New evidence 2017]	1B
23. ***It is suggested*** that given the increase in evidence of improved service user satisfaction and earlier functional independence, without adverse effects on dislocation rates when hip precautions are relaxed or discontinued, occupational therapists engage in local discussion/review of hip precaution protocols with their surgical and multidisciplinary teams. *(Barnsley et al 2015 [B]; Coole et al 2013 [C]; Drummond et al 2012 [C]; McQuaid et al 2014 [C]; O'Donnell et al 2006 [D]; Peak et al 2005 [B]; Restrepo et al 2011 [B]; Smith and Sackley 2016 [C]; Smith et al 2016 [A]; van der Weegen et al 2016 [B]; Ververeli et al 2009 [B])* [Statement amended, new evidence 2017]	2B

Hol et al (2010) carried out a systematic review to examine the evidence relating to partial versus unrestricted weight-bearing following total hip replacement (using an uncemented femoral stem). The 13 studies reviewed were not all randomised controlled trials and had relatively small sample sizes. Moderate to strong evidence was suggested, however, for full weight-bearing immediately post-operatively, with subsequent benefits of faster rehabilitation and return to functional independence. Despite the variation in methods, minimal risk of stem migration with full-weight bearing was indicated and the authors recommended early rehabilitation after uncemented total hip replacement. This evidence is valuable for occupational therapists to be aware of, but in relation to specific recommendations, practice will need to be guided by local surgical protocols and joint working with physiotherapists within the multidisciplinary team.

The evidence identified from the literature search specifically related to the requirement for hip precautions following total hip replacement was relatively limited and, at the time of the guideline review, there were few additional primary research studies, as highlighted by the more recent systematic reviews.

Smith et al (2016) conducted a Cochrane review to 'assess the effects of provision of assistive devices, education on hip precautions, environmental modifications and training in activities of daily living and extended activities of daily living' for individuals who had undergone a total hip replacement. Only two trials were included which focused on hip precautions, both of which were pre-2012 and, as such, were included in the original guideline as evidence **(Ververeli et al 2009, Peak et al 2005)**. The studies (discussed below), which were rated as low quality, meant that it was not possible to substantiate from the current evidence whether hip precautions (with or without the addition of equipment and functional restrictions) are actually effective in preventing dislocation or improving outcomes. A systematic review, undertaken by **Barnsley et al (2015)**, reviewed the same evidence but considered that the studies opened up the suggestion that the use of hip precautions did not improve dislocation rates and were associated with a slower return to activities, increased expense and decreased service user satisfaction.

The systematic review undertaken by **van der Weegen et al (2016)** included, in addition to the Ververeli et al and Peak et al studies, a further randomised controlled trial and three studies using a non-randomised trial design. The number of procedures and observed dislocations for the 1,084 participants were pooled (other data was too heterogeneous). Dislocation rates were compared on a number of variables, but the overall rates for the pooled 'restrictions' group (n=528) was 1.5% (n=8), compared to 1.0% (n=6) in the 'unrestricted' group. In the unrestricted (or 'less restrictive') group, resumption of activities was significantly better in four studies and length of stay significantly shorter in two studies. The authors highlight that there are many variables which influence the risk of dislocation post-operatively, but the evidence reviewed did not indicate a worse dislocation rate when protocols were in place for less restrictive or no precautions.

An American randomised controlled trial **(Peak et al 2005)** involved 265 service users and identified two groups: one 'restricted' and one 'unrestricted'. Both groups, who had undergone anterolateral approach surgery, were asked to limit their range of movement to less than 90 degrees of flexion and 45 degrees of external and internal rotation, and to avoid adduction for the first six weeks after the procedure. Service users in the restricted group were managed with the placement of an abduction pillow in the operating room before bed transfer and used pillows to maintain abduction while in bed. They also used elevated toilet seats and elevated chairs in the hospital, rehabilitation facility and at home, and were prevented from sleeping on their side, from driving and from being a passenger in a car. Service users in the unrestricted group were not *required* to follow additional restrictions, but could *choose* to use equipment if they wished for comfort. This choice gave rise to methodological concerns about the overlap in the intervention received by the study and control groups. The study was not strictly comparing 'precautions' against 'no precautions'. From the service user perspective, the results suggested that they were much more satisfied when fewer restrictions were imposed on them. Removal of restrictions resulted in lower costs and increased service user satisfaction, and earlier return to daily functions (better sleep, return to work earlier once able to drive). There was one dislocation in the entire cohort (prevalence 0.33%), that being in the restricted group, and it occurred during transfer from the operating table post-surgery.

Ververeli et al (2009) conducted a smaller, randomised controlled trial, again in America, which involved 81 service users undergoing anterolateral approach surgery. The study aimed to determine any differences between outcomes for the standard group (who were under the standard hip precautions utilised by this facility) and outcomes for the early rehabilitation group (who had relaxed precautions with the only restriction being not crossing their legs at the thighs). There were no dislocations and the relaxed precautions group were walking without a limp and driving earlier. The researchers concluded that the early rehabilitation protocol increased the pace of recovery compared to a pathway with hip precautions, without increasing complications.

The studies by Peak et al (2005) and Ververeli et al (2009) both focused on uncomplicated hip replacements and hip precautions were not fully removed. Methodological limitations mean that findings cannot be fully adopted or generalised and in both cases the evidence was downgraded from high to moderate to reflect potential for bias and some concerns regarding confidence in applicability of the findings.

Both these randomised controlled trials were included in a literature review of three studies that aimed to identify how necessary hip restrictions for avoiding dislocation were, following hemiarthroplasty or total hip replacement in older people with a hip fracture **(Stewart and McMillan 2011)**. In addition to the studies by Peak et al and Ververeli et al, Stewart and McMillan reviewed a study by Talbot, Brown and Treble reported in 2002. That study prospectively investigated primary total hip replacement via the anterolateral approach with no hip restrictions observed post-operatively. Stewart and McMillan noted that although the dislocation rate in this study was reported as low, at 0.6%, there was no control and follow-up was only for a period of six weeks.

Stewart and McMillan therefore concluded that there was insufficient evidence regarding how necessary hip precautions are for avoiding dislocation following total hip replacement. There did, however, appear to be a consensus that surgical approach, surgeon skill, cognitive capacity and hospital volume had greater importance in dislocation rates. Modifying hip precautions by reducing limitations seemed to demonstrate benefits for service users as reported by Peak et al (2005) and Ververeli et al (2009). Stewart and McMillan also identified a higher risk of dislocation post-fracture than for elective surgery, with implications that those who experience a fractured hip tend to be frailer and with co-morbidities, and therefore less generally fit and well than those receiving elective surgery.

The anterolateral or direct anterior approach was also the surgical technique used in a study by **Restrepo et al (2011)**. Restrepo et al evaluated the incidence of dislocation in a prospective cohort of 2,532 service users undergoing total hip replacement. This research involved a no-restriction protocol, such that there were no traditional functional restrictions applied post-operatively. Additionally, those with complications, such as a history of surgery on the contralateral hip or neuromuscular disease, were included. Restrepo et al reported four dislocations in the followed cohort of 2,386 service users (rate of 0.15%) and suggested that despite some study limitations, removal of hip restrictions did not increase the incidence of early dislocation using this approach.

A national survey of occupational therapy practice for hip precautions following primary total hip replacement identified that occupational therapists generally agree on the main movements that service users are advised to avoid following primary elective total hip replacement, namely not flexing the hip beyond 90 degrees, and avoiding adduction and internal/external rotation of the hip **(Drummond et al 2012)**. The length of time hip precautions were recommended to be observed varied, however, ranging from six weeks to over twelve weeks. The rationale for teaching hip precautions given by respondents was also varied and lacked consensus. The most common reported reason was surgical opinion, with occupational therapy policy and surgical approach the other most frequent responses. The authors highlighted that very few respondents identified an evidence base as the reason for precautions being applied.

A subsequent qualitative study by **Coole et al (2013)** further explored the practitioner's perspectives on hip precautions following total hip replacement. Barriers to moving away from routine hip precaution recommendations included: perceived risk of dislocation and impairment of tissue healing; fear of litigation; tradition; and lack of evidence that precautions should not be used. The authors established, however, that a relaxation of routine hip precautions was perceived as having the potential to impact on the recovery and satisfaction of the service user, the role and skill mix of therapy services, the use of resources and the length of hospital stay. An overriding message from practitioners was the need for a definitive trial which could provide evidence on the efficacy and outcomes of hip precautions.

Smith and Sackley (2016), building on the work by **Drummond et al (2012)**, explored the current practice of hip precautions and the provision of equipment by both occupational therapists and physiotherapists. Hip precaution advice was provided routinely by 97% of respondents, with advice about main movements to be avoided and variation in time periods recommended largely reflecting the findings of Drummond's earlier research. In the context of prescribing precautions, the main reasons identified were surgical and therapy protocols and the clinician's personal assessment; 48% of respondents identified, however, that they would like to change practice to become more individualised. This study confirms the variability in practice and that research is still required to determine the 'whether and to whom' in the context of providing equipment and recommending hip precautions post-total hip replacement.

A study **(McQuaid et al 2014)**, based on one service's revised orthopaedics pathway following a consultant-led decision to remove routine hip precautions, reported on the outcomes and influence on the occupational therapy service. Telephone interviews at 12 weeks post-surgery confirmed that 97.5% (n=78) of those receiving elective surgery had not used hip precautions. No rise in dislocation rate was identified. All service users had received an occupational therapy assessment, and of those 89% were provided with equipment to facilitate their independent and safe discharge, equipment which was used on average for a shorter period compared to when precautions were in place. The authors suggest that the new pathway was not detrimental and contributed to reduced length of stay. It was noted, however, that in the absence of routinely prescribed precautions and equipment, assessment and intervention demands high-level clinical reasoning by the occupational therapist.

While the two randomised controlled trials **(Peak et al 2005, Ververeli et al 2009)** and the prospective study **(Restrepo et al 2011)** provided insight into the potential benefits of reducing or removing hip precautions, occupational therapists work as members of the multidisciplinary team and therefore, given the current evidence of the importance of surgical expertise and approach in possible dislocation risk, and lack of research that investigates whether precautions are effective, it is not appropriate to develop specific hip restriction recommendations that can be implemented by all occupational therapists. It is, therefore, essential that therapists consult with the surgical team with whom they are working regarding any specific precautions to be followed post-operatively.

By sharp contrast in terms of study design, a descriptive case study report **(Malik et al 2002)** identified three cases where service users had dislocated post-operatively at home when turning to answer the telephone. While very low-level descriptive evidence, the report highlighted the importance of discussing hip precautions and the performance of basic daily living activities with service users; for example, placing a telephone in an easily accessible location and safe limb positioning as opposed to automatically turning to answer a call should be simple, low-risk advice.

The study by Malik et al highlights that irrespective of the level of hip precautions identified by a surgical team, occupational therapists can provide advice on appropriate positional behaviours. This facilitates good positioning and joint care and can be applicable whether specific restrictions are reduced or removed, or whether certain items of equipment are provided to meet individual need. It should be emphasised that there is always the risk that the service user will not follow precautions or advice and, therefore, an approach that encourages good joint positioning and care, while reinforcing any hip precaution protocols in place, is potentially more empowering to the service user.

The practice of hip precautions is changing in some areas and experts on the guideline development group, and subsequent guideline review group, were aware of the removal of hip restrictions in some UK institutions. Occupational therapists will, therefore, continue to find that the hip precaution protocols they are expected to reinforce and support will be variable dependent on where they are working. It is suggested that given the potential for emerging evidence from those services reducing their restrictions on the risks of dislocation, occupational therapists should ensure they are actively involved in discussing the implications of any changes in practice for occupational therapy intervention and service user outcomes.

The emerging evidence is that the prescription of hip precautions is being considered increasingly unnecessary and is likely to decrease. It is, therefore, essential that occupational therapists are up to date with the latest evidence base and actively contribute to and inform multidisciplinary discussion and future practice developments. An interesting article by **O'Donnell et al (2006)**, while very low evidence, offers a descriptive account of how a Canadian team examined the available evidence and undertook a consensus process to develop primary total hip replacement guidelines for their service. It is vital that occupational therapists proactively engage in the 'hip precautions debate', and O'Donnell et al's therapist-led/co-ordinated consensus project could provide useful information about how this process might be taken forward locally.

6.5 Enhanced recovery

Evidence overview – Enhanced recovery
The evidence specifically for occupational therapy post-operatively is limited. More generally, the evidence shows that the implementation of clinical pathways and enhanced recovery programmes can make a difference to length of hospital stay. However, one study noted that post-discharge challenges can still occur. Additionally, the evidence supports home-based rehabilitation in terms of reducing length of hospital stay, and multidisciplinary rehabilitation in terms of positive outcomes for service users and institutions.

6.5.1 Introduction

The period between admission and discharge for routine elective surgery has reduced in recent years, with a median length of stay recorded as four days for a cemented total hip replacement and three days for an uncemented total hip replacement in England during 2014/2015 (NHS Digital 2015). In Scotland, the average length of stay in 2015 was reported as 5.1 days (NHS National Services Scotland 2016).

Reducing the length of stay can potentially benefit the individual service user and the cost-effectiveness of service delivery. A procedure such as total hip replacement is relatively standardised and has, therefore, been appropriate for the focus of care pathway activity, particularly given that variations in the process of care can potentially be reduced. Care pathways, accelerated discharge and enhanced recovery programmes are common features of hip replacement interventions.

Clinical pathways should take into account national clinical guidelines that may influence intervention. A total hip replacement, for example, may be the intervention of choice for a hip fracture, and therefore relevant national guidelines for management of hip fracture should be cross-referenced (SIGN 2009, NICE 2011). There will also be many individual variables which contribute to or influence the length of stay which multidisciplinary teams will need to take into account. These may include, for example, living alone, medical issues post-operatively and the need for a care package on discharge **(Harte et al 2017)**.

6.5.2 Evidence

Enhanced recovery	
24. ***It is recommended*** that occupational therapists optimise length of stay, with due reference to care pathways and enhanced recovery programme guidance. *(Arshad et al 2014 [C]; Berend et al 2004 [C]; Bottros et al 2010 [C]; Brunenberg et al 2005 [C]; Husted et al 2008 [C]; Ibrahim et al 2013 [B]; Kim et al 2003 [B])* [New evidence 2017]	1B
25. ***It is recommended*** that the occupational therapist is involved in early multidisciplinary post-operative intervention for service users following hip replacement, providing either inpatient or home-based rehabilitation. *(Aasvang et al 2015 [D]; Ibrahim et al 2013 [B]; Iyengar et al 2007 [C]; Khan et al 2008 [A]; Pape et al 2013 [C]; Siggeirsdottir et al 2005 [C])* [New evidence 2017]	1A

A proportion of the literature reviewed made either direct or indirect references to length of hospital stay. This often focused on looking at potential individual service user factors and predictors (see section 6.1). The broader topic of clinical pathways and enhanced recovery programmes was also explored by some of the literature.

Kim et al (2003) undertook a critical review of evidence on clinical pathway effectiveness for total hip and knee replacement. All studies that reported on length of stay showed that with the implementation of clinical pathways, there were reductions in acute hospital length of stay and in hospital costs. Additionally, there were reduced or unchanged rates of complications and either improvement or no change in service user reported outcomes. There were, however, considerable variations within the 11 studies examined, with use of historical controls creating a potential for bias, hence interpretation should be cautious.

A defined joint recovery programme was examined in a Dutch low-level evidence case control study, which compared the cost-effectiveness for service users receiving the programme and those receiving usual care **(Brunenberg et al 2005)**. This also demonstrated a reduction in hospital length of stay and an improvement in joint and function that was statistically significant.

Bottros et al (2010) carried out a retrospective study that aimed to compare an enhanced recovery programme with a traditional approach. The study supported the enhanced recovery programme and emphasised the importance of the multidisciplinary team. There was no single factor identified as being responsible for reduced length of stay; however, influencing factors included surgical approach, pre-emptive and multimodal pre-operative analgesia, type of physical therapy, service user pre-habilitation and family education. A similar finding was determined from a study **(Berend et al 2004)** using a multimodal approach with pre- and post-operative education, 'aggressive' post-operative rehabilitation and attention to pre-emptive analgesia. This low-level retrospective study was reported with only very minimal information. On critical appraisal, the six-year period between data collection for the control (pre-programme) and study (post-programme) groups raised concerns about confounding variables and whether some change would have actually occurred because of the length of time between data collection. However, the study usefully confirmed that a significant reduction in length of stay could be achieved by focusing on the potential for change within a service.

Husted et al (2008) undertook a study to identify service user characteristics associated with length of stay in fast-track total hip and total knee replacement surgery. This prospective Danish study involved 712 service users and found that the mean length of stay was reduced from 8 to 3.8 days. The researchers therefore concluded that implementation of an accelerated programme was capable of leading to reductions in length of stay for unselected service users.

A more recent study, conducted by **Arshad et al (2014)**, compared the Norwich Enhanced Recovery Programme (NERP) with a non-enhanced programme, for both total hip and total knee replacements. The enhanced pre- and peri-operative multidisciplinary programme incorporated pain control, early intensive rehabilitation and the use of education to assist in the management of service user expectations. The focus of the research was on early clinical outcomes and safety. A shorter median length of stay was identified for those receiving the NERP, although this was not statistically significant and there was no significant change in any post-operative complications for that group.

The importance of a highly organised and structured multidisciplinary approach was reported as being particularly relevant for enhanced recovery and reduced length of stay in a review by **Ibrahim et al (2013)**, while **Pape et al (2013)** explored the impact of introducing a daily interprofessional meeting (to discuss barriers, discharge issues and make joint decisions) on length of stay for individuals following a total hip or total knee replacement. Using a case control study, the suggestion from Pape et al's research was that the length of stay for total hip replacement could potentially be significantly reduced (from a mean of 4.1 days to 2.7 days).

Clinical pathways are not used universally, but have demonstrated decreases in length of hospital stay. It is still essential, however, that an individual's needs, which can influence recovery, are taken into account within the context of a pathway. While the evidence on clinical pathways has not been occupational therapy-specific, occupational therapists need to be aware of pathways or programmes in place where they are working, and be clear about their contribution and role in optimising length of stay.

Intervention and rehabilitation post-operatively need to be instigated at the earliest opportunity given that the length of hospital stay may be only two to three days. A fast-track or enhanced programme can reduce length of stay, but there may also be post-discharge challenges such as limited physical function, post-operative pain, the use of analgesics or post-operative cognitive dysfunction, highlighting the need for 'optimal assessment' of post-operative function to guide rehabilitation **(Aasvang et al 2015)**.

Studies have investigated the role of targeted early rehabilitation provided at home in terms of influence on length of stay. **Iyengar et al (2007)** in a low-level prospective cohort study looked at home-based multidisciplinary rehabilitation following total hip replacement. Hospital stay was reduced without any increase in complication rates, although it should be noted that the service had a long baseline length of stay. **Siggeirsdottir et al (2005)** undertook a randomised controlled trial in which outcomes of service users who received pre-operative education/training and home-based rehabilitation were measured. This study had a number of limitations, including lack of information on the conventional treatment used as the control. It identified, however, that length of stay was shorter for the intervention group, and that additionally function and quality of life were enhanced compared to the conventional treatment.

A Cochrane review **(Khan et al 2008)** examined the evidence for effectiveness of organised multidisciplinary rehabilitation on activity and participation in adults following hip or knee replacement surgery for chronic arthropathy. Questions considered achievement of outcomes, the nature of the outcomes, and the influence and intensity of rehabilitation in relation to gains. While the high-quality review included five trials (619 participants), the studies themselves were highly heterogeneous and meta-analysis was therefore not feasible.

Occupational therapy-specific findings were not identified in the review and there were no studies that provided direct evidence that multidisciplinary rehabilitation following lower limb joint replacement achieved better outcomes compared with no treatment. There was evidence for the effectiveness of multidisciplinary rehabilitation in both inpatient and home-based settings, with 'silver' evidence that early and/or organised inpatient multidisciplinary rehabilitation led to more rapid attainment of functional milestones in the shorter term, as well as fewer post-operative complications, shorter hospital stay and reduced cost. However, there was no evidence that earlier inpatient rehabilitation improved participation. In relation to home-based multidisciplinary rehabilitation, there was 'silver'-level evidence for organised hospital at home care improving quality of life and disability in service users following hip replacement.

The duration of follow-up of service users after hip and knee replacement was limited to short and medium term (3–6 months post-operatively). It was not possible to determine whether gains made by participants in rehabilitation were maintained in the longer term (greater than 12 months). From this review, it was also not possible to suggest best 'dose' of therapy. Further studies are needed to suggest optimum number, duration and intensity of treatment sessions.

One study in the review produced 'silver'-level evidence for modest cost benefits arising from early inpatient rehabilitation. There was no good evidence, however, proving the overall cost-effectiveness of home-based programmes.

The review found there was modest support for hip replacement service users being assessed for their need for appropriate rehabilitative intervention. Assessment, it was suggested, could potentially be undertaken by any skilled member of the multidisciplinary team in order to maximise capacity for independent living and societal participation.

In summary, the Cochrane review identified evidence that multidisciplinary rehabilitation programmes could have a positive impact on service user-related outcomes, such as function and quality of life, as well as institutional outcomes, such as length of stay and cost. Additionally, the recommendations pertained to both early inpatient and home-based multidisciplinary rehabilitation programmes having benefit.

The literature search for the guideline review confirmed that evidence specifically relating to the nature of occupational therapy intervention immediately post-surgery remains very limited. Studies were more evident in the area of pre-operative intervention, and those that considered interventions in the inpatient environment took a broader 'rehabilitative' perspective. Post-operative occupational therapy intervention is normally based on the self-care, leisure and productivity needs and goals identified pre-operatively or on admission.

The ability of occupational therapy staff to provide early intervention, particularly if home-based, will be influenced by available resources.

6.6 Reduced demand on support services

Evidence overview – Reduced demand on support services
Research points to the presence of a level of stress experienced by carers of individuals awaiting total hip replacements, and while this did reduce post-surgery, it did not do so significantly. The evidence suggests carers should be considered when assessing service users, though occupational therapists will need to weigh this against the wishes of carers and service users.

6.6.1 Introduction

The outcome of reduced demand on support services focuses on encouraging the service user to do things they can usually do, or have the potential to manage independently, and not to unnecessarily rely on services for support. Occupational therapists, often in conjunction with social workers, will assess social considerations (i.e. ensuring adequate support in the community), liaising with the service user, informal carers and health and social care services if additional support is required.

In terms of what constitutes a support service, it is important that not only statutory services are considered. A significant amount of support is provided by informal carers, in the absence of whom there is the potential for increased demand on support services. It is acknowledged that there is considerable research available on carers within a wider context.

6.6.2 Evidence

Reduced demand on support services	
26. ***It is suggested*** that there are potential benefits in including informal carers in pre-operative assessment/education, and post-operative intervention, to maximise service user independence and reduce carer stress. *(Chow 2001 [C])*	2C

The literature search identified a lack of evidence that focused on support services on discharge and social considerations in the context of total hip replacement, despite pre-operative assessment of social support needs being essential to optimise length of stay through early discharge planning.

Individuals awaiting a total hip replacement will usually have experienced deteriorating physical function, increasing pain and stiffness, and, as such, this is likely to have had an impact on their functional abilities. **Chow (2001)**, in a UK study, investigated whether carers experienced stress from looking after individuals with osteoarthritis who were waiting for a total hip replacement. He found there was a degree of stress when caring for someone awaiting total hip replacement, with 91.3% of carers pre-operatively reporting some stress as measured by the Robinson Caregiver Strain Index. This had reduced by 23% post-surgery but was not found to be significant. The study was, however, small scale, had a proportion of drop-outs at the follow-up measures and some confounding factors. Additionally, while the study aimed to determine the impact of the intervention (surgery) on the outcome (caregiver stress), the post-operative period examined was only three months following the hip replacement.

The needs of carers should be taken into account when completing pre-operative assessments/interventions, involving them from the start, identifying needs and potential support requirements, and providing guidance and information about available resources. The study suggested that occupational therapists could run carers groups, teaching the skills and knowledge required in assisting service users in activities of daily living, stress management, problem-solving skills and reorganising the daily routine.

> *"It is vitally important that your relatives and carers are involved in pre-operation education – it's very easy to sit and be looked after and they are afraid they will do the wrong thing and damage the hip, so this can delay recovery. Where they are involved from the beginning they can encourage you to do the exercises and get going again."*
>
> *50+ Forum service user feedback (2012)*

Informal carers may choose not to be involved and the care receiver may also not want them to be directly involved. The dynamics around the caring relationship are often complex and the occupational therapist must be aware that this may impact on implementation of any recommendations. Opportunities to engage with carers should be offered, but may not be accepted.

The evidence suggested specific carers groups may be an option; however, the expert opinion on the guideline development group indicated that this is unlikely to be practicable in the immediate pre-operative and acute stages of intervention. Identifying potential carers could be feasible at the pre-operative assessment, but the logistics of subsequently organising a group would be complex and resource heavy. In the absence of specific evidence regarding carers groups in this clinical context, there is no indication that they would necessarily be any more effective than the involvement of informal carers individually in the pre-operative assessment/education and post-operative intervention. While there may be a barrier for occupational therapists to provide carers groups, they can ensure family members/carers are informed of support services in the local area that may be able to offer advice and support, and told of their right to a carer assessment. More formal opportunities for occupational therapy advice and contribution to carer education and support may be extremely pertinent earlier in the overall care pathway for arthritis.

6.7 Potential impact of the recommendations

6.7.1 Desired outcomes

Implementation of the recommendations has the potential to deliver some key outcomes for service users and services, most notably:

- Service users feel more prepared and less anxious about their surgery.
- Service users are satisfied with their individualised care that provides the tools needed to help them resume meaningful occupations post-surgery.
- Service users have an optimised post-operative length of stay in the hospital that provides the best start to recovery.
- Service users who would like to return to work are encouraged and feel enabled to do so.
- Post-operative care in the community is individualised and takes into account carers, service users and any potential carers.

6.7.2 Risk management

Implementation of the guideline recommendations must be in the context of effective risk assessment and risk management. Hip precautions are one area where risk management is necessary. While the evidence suggests that removing hip precautions does not result in more adverse effects than the use of hip precautions, the evidence overall is inconclusive. Hence the recommendations focus on ensuring individualised care that involves discussion with the multidisciplinary team.

6.7.3 Generalisability

The variation in study method and level has been taken into account in the development of the recommendations to ensure that findings have not been overgeneralised. The guideline development group utilised evidence that was felt to be generalisable to the UK target population.

6.7.4 Social determinants of health

The recommendations focusing on helping individuals to resume the occupations that are meaningful to them are important to enable the service user to return to a fulfilling lifestyle. As total hip replacement is performed on younger, often more active, service users, the 2017 review has highlighted the need to include return to work, sports and physical activity in these discussions.

7 Service user perspectives of the recommendations

7.1 Overall service user opinions

Service users involved in the consultation on outcomes for the first edition were given the opportunity of expressing an interest in further involvement in the project. Those individuals who intimated they would be willing to provide further information or would like to contribute more to the guideline development work being undertaken by the Royal College of Occupational Therapists Specialist Section – Trauma and Orthopaedics were subsequently contacted and asked whether they would be willing to review the draft recommendations.

In 2012, a facilitated meeting was offered to members of the Rushcliffe 50+ Forum Health Sub Group (two attended the meeting, one completed the consultation by post and one via a telephone discussion and subsequent completion of the questionnaire) and a postal consultation was carried out with those interested service users known to the Golden Jubilee National Hospital (responses returned by 23 out of 40 people contacted).

This consultation on the draft recommendations, in addition to any general comments, sought views on three key issues:

Key issue	'Yes' response
Do you think the recommendations are easy to understand?	85%
Do you think these recommendations will help service users prepare for their operation?	89%
Do you think these recommendations will help service users to achieve the benefits and outcomes they want after their surgery?	89%

A number of respondents provided remarks on each key issue, and 15 provided additional comments. Some of these comments have been incorporated in the relevant recommendation sections as service user feedback statements.

Service user perspectives on the changes from the review were sought via the contacts and social media presence of the National Rheumatoid Arthritis Society and Arthritis Care. Unfortunately no service users responded.

7.2 Understanding the recommendations

The majority of service users felt that they were able to understand the recommendation statements. This guideline's target audience is occupational therapy personnel and therefore the response that 85% of the service users indicated the recommendations were easy to understand was a positive outcome. It is appreciated that some respondents nonetheless found the language 'jargonistic', suggesting that if the target audience was service users, the language could be usefully reviewed.

"The recommendations are very clear and take you through the journey that you as a patient go on when having a planned hip replacement."

50+ Forum service user feedback (2012)

"The recommendations are a clear picture, to all patients and their relatives, to give them an understanding of the services available to them."

Golden Jubilee National Hospital service user feedback (2012)

A specific service user version of this guideline was not part of the guideline development project; however, the response received from service users does support the intention that the guideline may be of benefit to service users and carers, and potentially enable them to be better informed about the occupational therapy process (section 4.3).

7.3 Preparing for the operation and achieving benefits and outcomes after surgery

The views received by service users reviewing the draft recommendations highlighted the relevance of the statements in preparing service users for their operation, and in their contribution to enabling service users to achieve the benefits and outcomes they want after their surgery.

Respondents did not specifically comment on all recommendations, but feedback included common themes of the importance of being treated as an individual, receiving information and effective communication. These principles of practice should essentially underpin every recommendation.

"It is really important you are treated as an individual. In a group the information seems very generalised and you think, 'well my home or lifestyle isn't like that' so you don't necessarily get the benefit. But if someone talks and LISTENS to you then these recommendations will make a lot of difference."

50+ Forum service user feedback (2012)

"Being able to ask questions without feeling stupid is so important - everyone is different so some people will be worried about getting back to work - others will be thinking, how can I make a cup of tea in my tiny kitchen with a zimmer frame."

50+ Forum service user feedback (2012)

"Feeling like you matter as an individual cannot be underestimated - it really impacts on your belief you can do it and get back to normal."

50+ Forum service user feedback (2012)

"By recommending areas to be addressed pre-op, this will give patients an insight into what is best for their individual and collective needs."

Golden Jubilee National Hospital service user feedback (2012)

"Communication is of key importance both in pre-operative and post-operative education of the patient's wellbeing and I think the recommendations cover most aspects required."

Golden Jubilee National Hospital service user feedback (2012)

The objective of this guideline is to describe 'the most appropriate care or action to be taken by occupational therapists working with adults undergoing total hip replacement' (see section 3). Taking that objective in the context of the person-centred and holistic philosophy of occupational therapy, it is pertinent to conclude this section of the guideline document with a comment from a service user:

"By outlining the areas best served to promote the patient's wellbeing after surgery, it gives the patients more chance of achieving their post-op aims of maximum recovery."

Golden Jubilee National Hospital service user feedback (2012)

8 Implementation of the guideline

This practice guideline aims to support occupational therapists to take the most appropriate care or action when working with adults who are undergoing total hip replacement.

Familiarisation with the guideline document will be an important first step for both individual practitioners and their managers. It is, therefore, imperative that occupational therapists and managers working in this clinical area take responsibility to review the guideline recommendations within the context of their practice.

Bringing the guideline to the attention of colleagues within the multidisciplinary team and service commissioners should also be a priority.

A further action to facilitate implementation must be for lead therapists to consider the 'levers' and 'barriers' within their local organisation and culture that may have an impact on any changes that may be necessary to practice. Section 8.2 identifies some potential barriers that may be applicable, while section 8.3 provides details of resources to facilitate implementation.

8.1 Dissemination and promotion

Awareness and implementation of this practice guideline are important if it is to influence and have an impact on occupational therapy practice, and are therefore important not only for current practitioners but for occupational therapy students who are the future workforce.

To facilitate dissemination, the full practice guideline is available to download freely from the Royal College of Occupational Therapists' website.

The guideline has been promoted to its key target audience of occupational therapists and to relevant others using professional networks and publications, internet and social media channels.

8.2 Organisational and financial barriers

The recommendations stated within this guideline document are intended to facilitate occupational therapy staff to contribute effectively to service user-centred and service delivery-centred outcomes following total hip replacement. Service user-centred outcomes may be affected if the individual does not receive pre-operative assessment and education or early post-operative occupational therapy intervention.

It is recognised, however, that there will be potential barriers, both organisational and financial, which may influence application of the recommendations. It is important that occupational therapists take these into account when implementing this guideline.

The recommendations are varied and any specific organisational or financial barriers have been described within the relevant sections.

In terms of the overall most critical resource required to implement these guideline recommendations, this is undoubtedly the availability of occupational therapy personnel within the multidisciplinary team. Care pathways are underpinned by interdisciplinary working and appropriate skill mix within the team. While 'generic working' may be a driving force in some services, it is important to recognise the value and contribution of specific skills and the experience of different professions and bands of staff in delivering the various elements of the pathway. For example, an individualised comprehensive occupational therapy assessment requires the experience and knowledge of a skilled therapist, while a trained support worker can effectively deliver components of a standardised education programme.

Staffing resources will be important in facilitating implementation, particularly where there may be an increased throughput of service users receiving a total hip replacement or introduction of a seven-day service within an ongoing climate of cost efficiencies.

In particular, occupational therapy personnel may be faced with implementing recommendations within the context of elective services that are constantly changing, with the drive for enhanced recovery programmes aiming to decrease length of stay and providing earlier rehabilitation. This can mean providing intervention for service users who feel less prepared for surgery, who have less time to recover on the ward, and where there is less time for the multidisciplinary team to arrange plans post-operatively.

The variations in service focus and in resources available within the community, particularly post-surgical rehabilitation options and equipment provision, may also result in challenges to implementing the recommendations without compromising care. This may be relevant for those recommendations which focus on holistic assessment and intervention, and those which also address longer-term goals for the service user.

8.3 Implementation resources

Three core implementation resources are available to support this practice guideline. All implementation resources can be downloaded, together with the full guideline document, from the publications section (Practice guidelines) of the Royal College of Occupational Therapists' website.

8.3.1 Quick reference guide

The quick reference guide lists the recommendations and indicates their strength and the quality of the evidence leading to their development.

This is intended to be used by practitioners as an easily accessible reminder of the recommendations for Intervention. It should ideally be used once the practitioner has read the full guideline document. This is important to ensure an appreciation and understanding of how the recommendations were developed and their context.

The quick reference guide includes the following:

- Introduction.
- List of the recommendations, their strength, and the quality of the evidence leading to their development.
- Evidence overview.
- Outline of context and occupational therapy role.

8.3.2 Audit form

It is recommended that occupational therapists use the Royal College of Occupational Therapists' audit form that supports this guideline.

The audit form for this guideline provides a template for individual occupational therapists or services to audit and review their current interventions against the recommendations. The aim is to encourage a reflection on current practice and to consider, where this does not follow the recommendations, the clinical reasoning in place to support decisions.

A baseline assessment conducted using the audit form can be repeated to enable review of progress on actions identified from the audit. It can be useful to undertake a routine audit every one or two years to monitor ongoing compliance.

The audit form, while initially providing a tool for use within an individual/service context, offers the potential for future benchmarking and wider comparative analysis.

8.3.3 Continuing professional development/knowledge transfer resource

The continuing professional development resource is interactive and can be tailored for local use. The session can be used for group or self-directed learning, or for raising awareness of the guideline at multidisciplinary meetings, study days or events.

A feedback form is also available to provide comment on the guideline and implementation resources to the Royal College of Occupational Therapists.

8.3.4 Other associated resources

Additional resources available include:

- Occupational therapy evidence fact sheet.
- Implementation tips.

Accessing the implementation resources

The quick reference guide, audit form and continuing professional development session resources are available as separate documents.

These can be downloaded, together with the full guideline document, from the publications section (Practice guidelines) of the Royal College of Occupational Therapists' website: *www.rcot.co.uk/practice-resources/rcot-publications/member/practice-guidelines-publications.*

The resources can also be accessed via the webpages of the Royal College of Occupational Therapists Specialist Section – Trauma and Orthopaedics.

9 Recommendations for future research

The review of the evidence identified a lack of occupational therapy primary research specific to occupational therapy and total hip replacement.

The effectiveness of occupation-focused interventions continues to be the major priority identified by occupational therapists for research activity.' Establishing that effectiveness is closely linked to the use of standardised assessments and outcome measures in the provision of services, and to cost-effectiveness studies which support the commissioning of occupation-focused services (COT 2007, p12).

The evidence reviewed for both the first and second editions of the guideline has clearly identified a priority for further high-quality clinical trials in relation to occupational therapy and the impact of relaxing hip precautions on rehabilitation outcomes and dislocation rates (Drummond et al 2012). As researchers and clinicians explore the removal of hip precautions, the impact should be audited and published for future consideration.

The guideline development group additionally recommends a number of potential topics where further research could be focused.

Outcome measures in the acute setting:

- The need for an appropriate standardised assessment and outcome measure for acute, fast-tracked rehabilitation post-total hip replacement, in the context that the National Institute for Health and Clinical Excellence is recommending home-based over bed based rehabilitation (NICE 2011).
- An outcome measure that extends beyond the acute stage and into the community, which can promote a seamless rehabilitation programme that builds on achievement without unnecessary duplication.

Role in work and employment-related interventions:

- Interventions aimed at enabling service users to maintain work roles while waiting for surgery.
- The effectiveness of community-based services that facilitate return to work for those in employment prior to surgery and the unemployed.
- Research is currently being undertaken to investigate the use of Intervention Mapping in designing an intervention occupational therapists can use to assist service users in returning to work (Coole et al 2016).

Focus on complex needs and occupational therapy intervention:

- Use of outcome measures and intensive rehabilitation programmes post-operatively, either inpatient or at home with full support.

ɐ effect of comprehensive pre-operative assessment, home visits and care ɪnagement planning prior to surgery on service user and service outcomes.

Otııer:

- The occupational therapy role in pain management.
- What service users and carers particularly value in the delivery of the occupational therapy service.
- The occupational therapy role in standardised care pathways following total hip replacement.
- The impact of acute interventions on levels of dependency and the need for services to support discharge.
- Models of service delivery including the effectiveness of seven-day working.
- The job roles and responsibilities for qualified compared to unqualified staff in the delivery of occupational therapy for adults undergoing total hip replacement.
- The role of occupational therapists in enabling increased physical activity and/or return to sports following total hip replacement.
- The role of occupational therapists in assisting with social reintegration (identified in Smith et al 2016).

10 Guideline development process

Sections 10 and 11 provide the details of the development process and methodology for the first edition of the guideline. Section 12 outlines the various elements of the process for the review and update for this second edition. Detailed information on the steps of the guideline development and review processes can be found in the *Practice guideline development manual 3rd edition* (COT 2017a).

10.1 The guideline development group

The membership of the core guideline development group (see Appendix 1 for full list) comprised six occupational therapists with expertise and experience in the field of orthopaedics and/or older people. It was determined that given the very specific occupational therapy nature of this practice guideline, the core group would be profession specific, with the expertise required from other stakeholders and service users most effectively obtained outside of core group meetings, via a reference group and consultation.

The core group members were all practising therapists, undertaking the guideline development work mainly in their private time, with support from employers to attend meetings. To facilitate the progress of the guideline development, much of the liaison and activity undertaken by group members was therefore carried out at a distance, using email correspondence to effect communications.

Two members of the Royal College of Occupational Therapists' Research and Development Team were co-opted as additional critical appraisers. The Research and Development Manager at the College was also co-opted to take on the role of editorial lead.

10.2 Stakeholder involvement

Stakeholders with a potential interest in the guideline development were identified by the core group membership at the preliminary guideline meeting. Specific attention was given to identifying professional colleagues who may be working as part of the multidisciplinary team and national voluntary organisations that may represent service users.

Identified stakeholders were subsequently contacted and invited to comment on a draft scope document. Feedback was reviewed and, where indicated, incorporated into the final scope document, which was then submitted to the Royal College of Occupational Therapists' Practice Publications Group for approval.

Stakeholders who expressed an interest in remaining involved became the virtual guideline development stakeholder reference group. The members of this group represented professional bodies and clinical experts within medicine, nursing, physiotherapy and social work as follows:

- Royal College of Surgeons of England
- British Hip Society

- Royal College of Nursing
- British Association of Social Work
- Chartered Society of Physiotherapy

The full draft guideline document was sent to each of the stakeholder reference group representatives for their review. All comments were duly considered for inclusion within the final guideline document.

10.3 Service user involvement

The guideline development group identified that obtaining service user perspectives was vital to the project, but it was highlighted immediately that there was no easily identifiable forum to facilitate this involvement. The occupational therapist's contact with service users receiving a total hip replacement and their carers is normally time limited by the nature of the condition and short-term occupational therapy intervention. As such, identification of service users to be involved in the guideline project was practically difficult. Two forums were, however, known to the guideline development group, from whom it would be feasible to request involvement from service user representatives, namely the Golden Jubilee National Hospital in Scotland and the Rushcliffe 50+ Forum Health Sub Group.

The guideline development group recognised that these groups would not necessarily be representative of all individuals undergoing total hip replacement, in terms of experiences, and cultural and ethnic diversity; however, as the national waiting times centre for Scotland, the Golden Jubilee National Hospital treats service users from across Scotland and, as such, has a diverse population representative of individuals from the Scottish Borders to the Highlands and Islands. The group, therefore, determined that individuals from the identified populations could take on a valuable role in the guideline development process, particularly in terms of their experiences as expert service users.

Group members decided that a significant contribution to the guideline development could be ascertained by consulting service user views via two core avenues:

- Service user perspectives on the importance of the service user-centred and service delivery-centred outcomes identified within the scope (section 4.1).
- Service user comments on the draft recommendations.

Details of the service user consultation on the outcomes are provided in Appendix 3.

The overall response rate and number of individual comments suggested service users were keen to share their perspectives of what was important to them following total hip replacement. The consultation demonstrated the high level of importance service users placed on functional independence, reduction of anxiety and the ability to resume their roles. The order of priority for the remaining outcomes, from highest to lowest, was low readmission rates, decreased length of hospital stay (term amended to enhanced recovery in this 2nd edition of the guideline), reduced demand on support services and, finally, reintegration into the community. It was decided by the guideline development group that presentation of the recommendations within this guideline document would reflect the order of prioritisation identified from the service user consultation (Appendix 3).

Service users involved in the consultation on outcomes were also given the opportunity of expressing an interest in further involvement in the project. Those individuals who intimated they would be willing to provide further information or would like to contribute more to the guideline development work being undertaken by the Royal College of Occupational Therapists Specialist Section – Trauma and Orthopaedics were subsequently contacted and asked whether they would be willing to review the draft recommendations.

A facilitated meeting was offered to members of the Rushcliffe 50+ Forum Health Sub Group and a postal consultation carried out with those interested service users known to the Golden Jubilee National Hospital. This consultation on the draft recommendations, in addition to any general comments, sought views on three key issues:

- Do you think the recommendations are easy to understand?
- Do you think these recommendations will help service users prepare for their operation?
- Do you think these recommendations will help service users to achieve the benefits and outcomes they want after their surgery?

All comments received were duly considered for inclusion within the final guideline document (section 7). Qualitative feedback from service users has been quoted alongside the recommendations where applicable. This approach aims to enhance the user perspective as an adjunct to the published evidence.

10.4 External peer review and consultation

Two independent peer reviewers were identified by the guideline development group to review a draft of the full guideline document. Reviewers were selected for their clinical expertise in the field and/or their guideline development experience or knowledge.

A one-month consultation period was established to enable members of the Royal College of Occupational Therapists Specialist Section – Trauma and Orthopaedics and Older People's Specialist Section (guideline end users) to comment on a draft of the full guideline. This consultation was also open to all members of the British Association of Occupational Therapists via the College's website.

The guideline development group considered the feedback received from all stakeholders, service users, peer reviewers and end users when finalising the recommendations and guideline document.

10.5 Conflict of interest

All guideline development group members (core group and co-opted), stakeholders and external peer reviewers were asked to declare any pecuniary or non-pecuniary conflict of interest, in line with the guideline development procedures (COT 2017a).

The nature of the potential or actual conflicts, made in the declarations (see Appendix 4), was not determined as being a risk to the transparency or impartiality of the guideline development.

10.6 Declaration of funding for the guideline development

This practice guideline for *Occupational therapy for adults undergoing total hip replacement* has been developed by a group led by a Specialist Section of the Royal College of Occupational Therapists. Specialist Sections are official branches of the College with specialist or regional interests, which, through their membership, are able to engage expert practitioners, educators and researchers in the development of guidelines and access the required clinical and research expertise.

As a membership organisation, the major source of funding for the Royal College of Occupational Therapists and its Specialist Sections is obtained from membership. Other sources of income are primarily from advertising and events.

The development and publication of this practice guideline was funded by the Royal College of Occupational Therapists and the Royal College of Occupational Therapists Specialist Section - Trauma and Orthopaedics.

The Royal College of Occupational Therapists provided specific resources to cover travel expenses, literature search, editorial and publication support.

Funding was also allocated and approved by the National Executive Committee of the Royal College of Occupational Therapists Specialist Section - Trauma and Orthopaedics to cover costs associated with sourcing copies of published articles, administration and promotional costs for the guideline development and its dissemination.

There were no external sources of funding.

Although the editorial lead was a member of staff at the Royal College of Occupational Therapists, the recommendation decisions were made by the guideline development group, and the views of the Royal College of Occupational Therapists have, therefore, not influenced the final recommendations within this guideline.

10.7 College appraisal and ratification process

The guideline proposal, scope and draft of the first edition were all reviewed and subsequently ratified by the Royal College of Occupational Therapists' Practice Publications Group, in line with the requirements of the 2nd edition of the *Practice guideline development manual* (COT 2011).

The first edition of this guideline was approved by the Practice Publications Group in July 2012.

The guideline review process commenced in September 2015 and this 2nd edition was approved by the Practice Publications Group in July 2017.

11 Guideline methodology

11.1 Guideline question

What evidence is there to support occupational therapy intervention with adults over the age of 18 undergoing total hip replacement?

The PICO (patient/population/problem, intervention, comparison and outcome) framework (Richardson et al 1995) was used to assist in developing the practice question further (see Table 1).

This approach clarifies the specific care group or condition being studied and the nature of the intervention to be investigated. A comparative treatment can be defined, where applicable, together with the anticipated outcomes (the desired/undesired or expected results of the intervention). This level of specificity is important in developing the question so that it addresses the requirements of the scope (College of Occupational Therapists 2017a).

Table 1: PICO framework

Patient (service user), **P**opulation or **P**roblem/circumstance	Adults, 18 years and over who undergo a total hip replacement
Intervention under investigation or action	Occupational therapy
Comparison, which is an alternative intervention or action	None
Outcome desired	Reduced anxiety. Maximised functional independence. Reduced demand on services. Resumption of roles. Reintegration into community. Decreased length of hospital stay. Low readmission rates.

11.2 Literature search strategy and outcomes

The literature search was carried out by a Royal College of Occupational Therapists' librarian, an expert in the field of occupational therapy literature, using a search strategy defined following discussion and agreement with the guideline development group.

The varied clinical and academic experience of the guideline development group meant that there was prior knowledge that the occupational therapy-specific evidence was likely to be limited. On the basis of this, the search covered a wide remit to ensure that there was adequate sensitivity to locating any relevant articles of which the group may not be aware.

11.2.1 Key terms

The strategy involved combining concept groups of key words. Eight key categories or concepts and their related terms were identified: hip operation, activities of daily living, home environment, client engagement, care pathways, multiple pathology, outcomes and occupational therapy (Appendix 5, Table A3).

Specific exclusions identified were: material published pre-2001, children/under 18 years of age, grey literature, language other than English (due to lack of resources for translation), hemiarthroplasty and animal surgery.

11.2.2 Databases

The databases searched reflected the most likely sources of published peer-reviewed occupational therapy and total hip replacement surgery evidence. Six core databases were searched from 2001 to the date the search was carried out (2011) as detailed in Table 2.

Table 2: Database searches

Core databases	Library search date
(CINAHL)	18/08/11
Medline	08/09/11
Allied and Complementary Medicine (AMED)	14/09/11
PsycINFO	15/09/11
Social Policy and Practice	16/09/11
Health Management Information Consortium (HMIC)	16/09/11

Five specialist databases were also searched: OTDBASE, OT SEARCH, OTseeker, NHS Economic Evaluation Database (NHS EED) and the Cochrane Library of systematic reviews and clinical trials (search date 19/09/11).

In the majority of cases, title, subject heading and abstracts were searched. Where the search term combinations were more general, some limitations were then applied to provide a stronger focus on relevance. Specific search fields and search result numbers are detailed in Appendix 5 (Tables A4 and A5).

Full search histories are available on request from the Royal College of Occupational Therapists.

11.2.3 Search results

The search findings identified a total of 3,647 results. These were scrutinised for duplicates, within database searches and cross-database search returns, by the Royal

College of Occupational Therapists' Research and Development Manager. The unique results lists were provided to the project group in addition to the original search lists. A total of 1,506 duplicates were removed.

11.3 Criteria for inclusion and exclusion of evidence

The resultant 2,141 search findings (title, keywords and abstracts) were screened by two members of the guideline development group against an eligibility checklist with the following inclusion and exclusion criteria:

Inclusion:

- Adult (18 years and over).
- Total hip replacement – either elective or following trauma.
- Rehabilitation or occupational therapy intervention discussed.
- Outcomes discussed (service user or service delivery related).

Exclusion:

- Primary focus on hip fracture.
- Cultural/health system/service delivery specific.
- Intervention specific (e.g. uni-professional [not occupational therapy], surgical or anaesthetic based).

This process enabled the identification of abstracts that would be potentially relevant to the practice guideline and should therefore be included within the critical appraisal process.

Following the screening, 2,038 items were excluded, resulting in a total of 103 items identified for full paper review and critical appraisal. Subsequent to the date of the literature search by the library, the guideline development group were alerted via their professional networks to two additional and pertinent publications. These met the inclusion criteria and were therefore critically appraised.

A total of 105 articles were, therefore, critically appraised and information compiled into evidence tables (Appendix 7), and 54 items of evidence were subsequently used to develop the recommendations (section 6).

An overview of the literature search outcomes is provided in Figure 1.

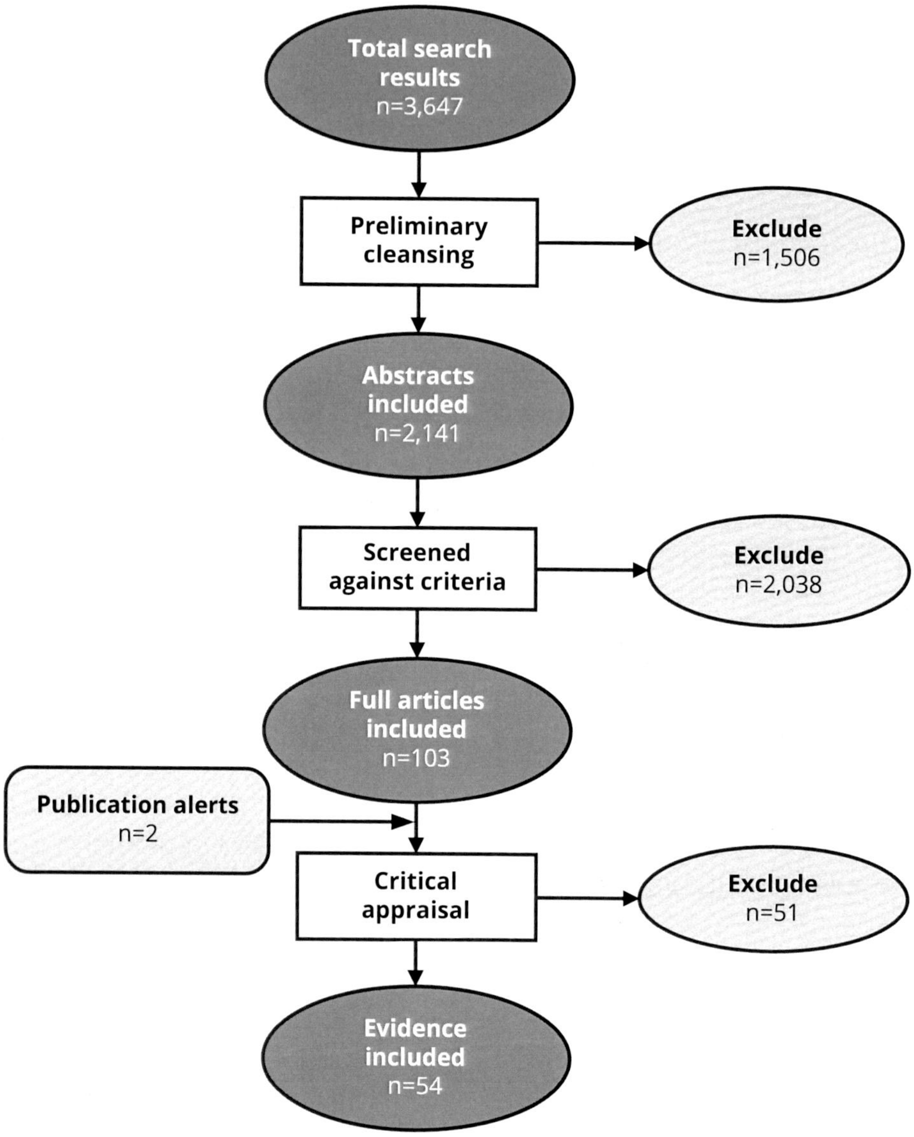

Figure 1 Literature search outcomes

11.4 Strengths and limitations of body of evidence

The 105 articles identified as potential evidence were independently reviewed by two members of the guideline development group/co-opted members. Any discrepancy in grading was resolved by a third reviewer.

The quality of the evidence was initially assessed using the Critical Appraisal Skills Programme (CASP) checklists (CASP 2010). Assessment took into account factors such as the appropriateness of the study design and recruitment strategy, procedural rigour in data collection and analysis, confounding factors and potential biases, transferability, precision of results and the value of the findings.

A grade was then also assigned to the evidence within an individual article using the GRADE approach as defined within the *Practice guidelines development manual 3rd edition* (COT 2017a). The grading reflects the research design and the confidence in the research findings.

The initial grading was allocated as follows:

- Randomised trial/systematic review = High
- Observational study = Low
- Any other evidence = Very Low

Limitations in the design of a study or its implementation may, however, bias the estimates of the treatment effect. If there were serious limitations, then the downgrading of the quality of the evidence was considered, using the criteria shown in Table 3.

Table 3: Grading evidence up or down (after GRADE Working Group 2004)

Decrease* grade if * Each quality criterion can reduce the quality by one or, if very serious, by two levels	• Serious or very serious limitation to study quality. • Important inconsistencies in results. • Some or major uncertainty about directness of the evidence. • Imprecise or sparse data (relatively few participants and/or events). • High probability of reporting bias.
Increase grade if	• Magnitude of the treatment effect is very large and consistent. • Evidence of a large dose–response relation. • All plausible confounders/biases would have decreased the magnitude of an apparent treatment effect. *Only studies with no major threats to validity should be upgraded.*

A decision to increase or decrease the initial grade of the evidence was justified in the evidence table. The 'moderate' category came into play if there was a suggested change in the grading. Evidence was ultimately graded in one of four categories, as detailed in Table 4. If there was no reason to up- or downgrade the evidence, then the original grading remained.

Once the methodological quality of each piece of evidence was assessed, details for each item of evidence were collated into an evidence table (Appendix 7).

Table 4: GRADE quality of evidence grading (after GRADE Working Group 2004)

Quality of evidence	Grading	Characteristics	Confidence
High	Grade A	Based on consistent results from well-performed randomised controlled trials, or overwhelming evidence of an alternative source, e.g. well-executed observational studies with strong effects.	True effect lies close to that of the estimate of the effect. Further research is very unlikely to change confidence in the estimate of the effect.
Moderate	Grade B	Based on randomised controlled trials where there are serious flaws in conduct, inconsistency, indirectness, imprecise estimates, reporting bias or some other combination of these limitations, or from other study designs with special strengths.	True effect likely to be close to the estimate of the effect but the possibility that there could be a substantial difference. Further research is likely to have an important impact on our confidence in the estimate of effect and may change the estimate.
Low	Grade C	Based on observational evidence, or from controlled trials with several very serious limitations.	True effect may be substantially different from the estimate of the effect. Further research is very likely to have an important impact on confidence in the estimate of the effect and is likely to change the estimate.
Very Low	Grade D	Based on case studies or expert opinion.	Any estimate of effect is very uncertain and may be far from the true effect.

11.5 Method used to arrive at recommendations

The evidence tables were used by the guideline development group as the basis to evaluate and judge each item's potential contribution to the development of the guideline recommendations.

The seven service user-centred and service delivery-centred outcomes (section 4.1) were used as the starting point, with identification of the relevant evidence in relation to each outcome. Where evidence was identified to support an outcome, this was reviewed. Each individual group member contributed their expert views to the discussion to develop recommendation options.

Where a number of items of evidence supported an identified outcome and subsequent recommendation, an overall quality of evidence rating was identified:

- Where the evidence outcomes pointed in different directions towards benefit and towards harm, the lowest quality of evidence determined the overall quality of evidence.

- Where the outcomes pointed in the same direction towards either benefit or harm, then the highest quality of evidence was appropriate to recommend an intervention and determined the overall quality of evidence.
- In circumstances where the balance of benefits and harm was uncertain, then the lowest grade of quality of evidence was assigned.

Strength of recommendation was the second element of the GRADE system applied using the College's categories, strong or conditional, to reflect the strength (Table 5).

Table 5: Strength of grade (after Guyatt et al 2008)

Strength	Grade	Benefits and risks	Implications
Strong	**1** ***'It is recommended. . .'***	Benefits appear to outweigh the risks (or vice versa) for the majority of the target group.	Most service users would want or should receive this course of intervention or action.
Conditional	**2** ***'It is suggested. . .'***	Risks and benefits are more closely balanced or there is more uncertainty in likely service user values and preferences.	The majority of service users would want this intervention but not all and therefore they should be supported to arrive at a decision for intervention consistent with the benefits and their values and preferences.

The development of the recommendations, including assignment of the overall quality and strength grading, was a consensus opinion obtained at the guideline development group meeting. There were no recommendations which were not agreed by all members so that no formal voting system or use of the nominal group technique was required. Fifty-four items of evidence were used to develop the recommendations.

A recommendation decision form was completed for each recommendation developed, recording key information about the evidence used to form the basis of that recommendation and the overall allocation of quality of evidence and strength of recommendation (recommendation decision forms are available on request from the Royal College of Occupational Therapists). The recommendation decision form facilitated discussion and recording of any specific or associated risks and benefits, and this was also highlighted in the final recommendation strength. Any judgement by the guideline development group was documented as part of this decision-making process.

12 Guideline review process

The guideline review followed a scheduled review process as outlined in the *Practice guideline development manual* (COT 2017a, section 3.15); this commenced three years after publication of the guideline.

The guideline question, objective and scope were unchanged, as were the criteria for inclusion or exclusion of evidence. This section outlines the process followed and, where necessary, cross-references to the original development process and methodology.

12.1 Guideline review group established

The review group consisted of two members of the original guideline development group and two new members, who were also members of the Royal College of Occupational Therapists Specialist Section – Trauma and Orthopaedics. All were occupational therapists with expertise and specialist interest in total hip replacement. Conflicts of interest were declared in line with the guideline development process requirements.

12.2 Identification of new evidence

A literature search was undertaken by the College's Library and Information Service. The scope was unchanged but the search strategy for the review was a refinement of the original strategy, as advised by the Library's information specialists, in order to increase the specificity and, as such, reduce the number of results which were inadvertently outside of the scope.

12.2.1 Key search terms

The strategy involved combining groups of search terms from five categories or concepts and their related terms: hip terms, generic occupational therapy-related terms, desired outcomes and finance/value terms (Appendix 6 Table A6).

12.2.2 Databases

Core and specialist databases were searched from the latest date of the guideline original search (1 January 2011) to November 2015.

The databases accessed were: EBSCOHOST platform (MEDLINE, CINAHL); OVID platform (AMED, HMIC, PsycINFO, Social Policy and Practice); OTseeker; OTDBASE; OT SEARCH; Cochrane Library; RCOT Library online catalogue; and hand searches of NICE and SIGN guidelines.

Details for the specific database searches (including period of search) are provided in Appendix 6 Tables A7 and A8.

12.2.3 Search results

The core and specialist searches produced a total of 605 results (EBSCOHOST platform n=465; OVID platform n=8 and specialist databases n=132). These were scrutinised for duplicates and anomalies by a College officer both within database and cross-database search findings. As a result of cleansing, 374 abstracts were returned for screening.

12.2.4 Screening and appraisal of evidence

Each of the 374 abstracts was screened by two members of the guideline review group against criteria identified in the guideline development process (sections 11.2.1, 11.3). This resulted in 254 items being excluded and 120 items of evidence being selected for independent appraisal by two group members. Two items subsequently screened in via publication alerts, between May 2016 and the guideline development group meeting held in September 2016, were also appraised. During the appraisal process, 94 articles were identified as inappropriate because they were out of scope.

An overview of the literature search outcomes is provided in Figure 2.

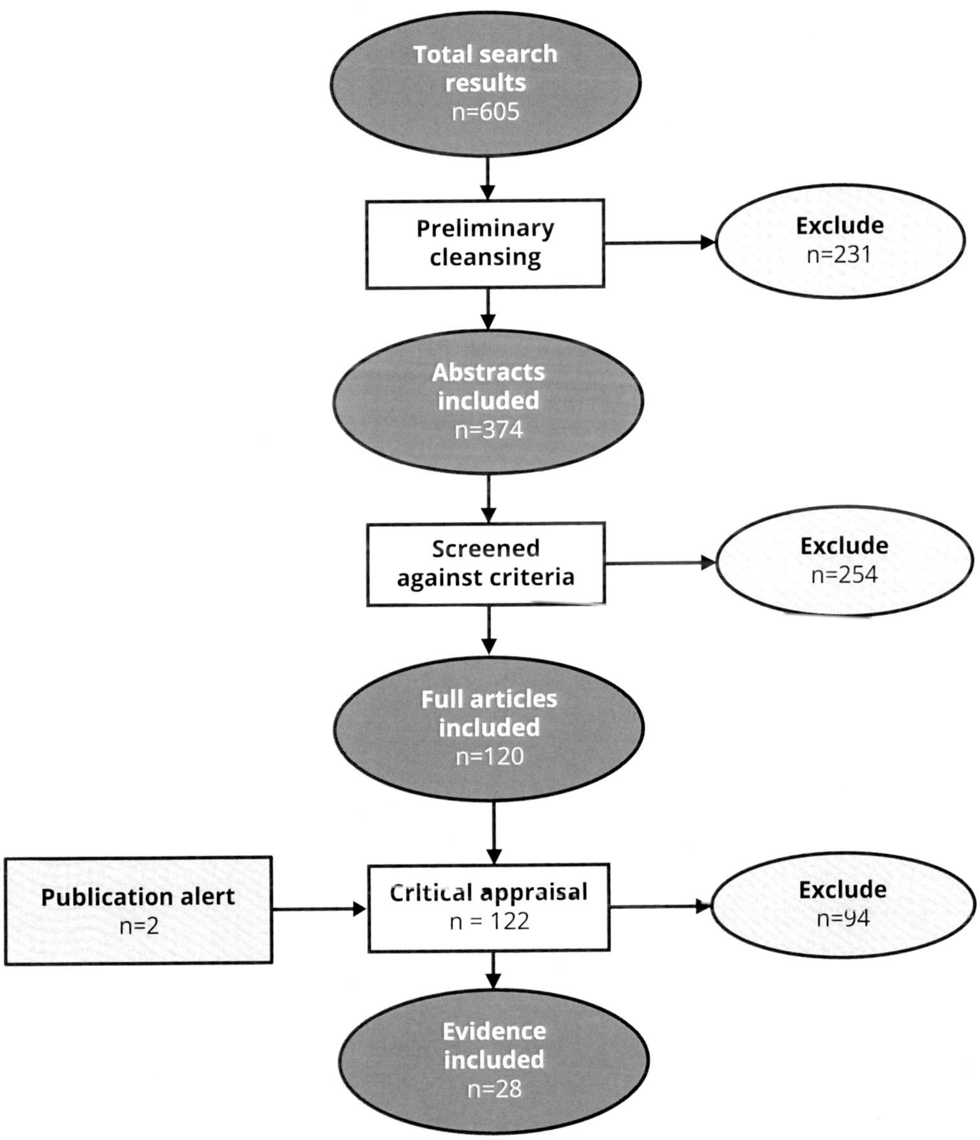

Figure 2 Review literature search outcomes

12.3 Assessment of update requirements

The review group discussions focused on:

- New evidence appraised.
- Consideration of any original material that was no longer appropriate and how this might need to be superseded or withdrawn.
- Consideration of any relevant feedback and comments received since the publication of the guideline.
- Development of recommendations where indicated by new evidence or knowledge.

The review group identified that there was some new evidence that was directly relevant to the guideline scope.

A total of 28 articles was agreed by consensus as being suitable for inclusion in an update of the guideline. These provided additional evidence to support 15 existing recommendation statements, minor amendments to two of those existing recommendation statements and the development of an additional recommendation.

Recommendation decision forms were completed and the group agreed, by consensus, that the grading of the new items of evidence did not affect the strength or grade of the original recommendations.

The 28 items of evidence were mostly graded as Low (Grade C, n=16), with six graded as Moderate (B), three graded High (A) and three graded Very Low (D).

12.4 External review

The additional evidence was mainly used to support existing recommendations, with one new recommendation and two revised recommendations. The engagement of stakeholders and service users focused on a consultation of the revised draft guideline for a month, mid-March to mid-April 2017. Where permission was obtained, those who participated are listed in the acknowledgements in Appendix 2.

End users: the draft updated guideline was made available to occupational therapists, particularly members of the College's Specialist Section – Trauma and Orthopaedics. All members were alerted via the professional body's magazine *OTnews* and website.

Stakeholders: stakeholders who had been invited to participate in the original consultation were contacted and invited to provide any comments on the full updated version of the guideline.

Service users: Arthritis Care and the National Rheumatoid Arthritis Society agreed to promote the opportunity for service users and lay individuals to contribute to the consultation of the draft of the 2nd edition of the guideline via their established networks and/or social media.

Peer review: two peer reviewers, experienced in both the topic and research, were identified to carry out an independent peer review of the updated draft.

12.5 College appraisal and ratification process

A draft of the 2nd edition of the guideline was submitted to the College's Practice Publications Group for review and approval in August 2017.

12.6 Overview of limitations and any potential bias of the guideline

Evidence included in the development of the guideline recommendations was sourced from published, peer-reviewed journal articles. Relevant policy documents have been referenced within the contextual information where applicable, but it is acknowledged that any key grey literature has not been included in the evidence.

The literature search identified limited primary research specific to occupational therapy and total hip replacement interventions. There was, however, a body of occupational therapy evidence which was relevant to the outcome of reducing anxiety, and particularly pre-operative intervention.

No evidence was identified which specifically addressed economic evaluation of occupational therapy for adults undergoing total hip replacement.

Evidence was frequently medically orientated or multidisciplinary, and a prominent topic was the investigation of service user-reported outcome measures. A number of studies investigated total hip and total knee replacements together, with findings from the two procedures not always being fully differentiated.

The review of the literature for the first and second editions combined identified 82 items of evidence from which recommendations were developed. The majority of this evidence was assessed as low grade (C) and was made up of predominantly cohort and qualitative studies:

Grade A = 6.1% (5)

Grade B = 19.7% (16)

Grade C = 61.7% (50)

Grade D = 13.5% (11)

The evidence did provide a number of higher-quality studies from a design and methodological perspective. The guideline group downgraded a proportion of the potential grade A studies due to concerns over the confidence of the estimate of the effect of the research. Systematic reviews were mainly graded as A or B, which was based on the robustness of the review methodology and reported outcomes. This did not necessarily reflect, however, the quality of the individual studies included within the review.

The decisions, and details on specific limitations of individual studies, are noted in the evidence tables in Appendix 7.

Table 6: Summary of evidence used to develop the recommendations

Category	Author	Year	Evidence quality
Maximised functional independence	Alviar et al	2011	B
	Berge et al	2004	B
	Vincent et al	2012	B
	Caracciolo and Giaquinto	2005	C
	Drummond et al	2013	C
	Fielden et al	2003	C
	Gillen et al	2007	C
	Hobbs et al	2011	C
	Johansson et al	2010	C
	Judge et al	2011	C
	Keifer and Emery	2004	C
	Lin and Kaplan	2004	C
	Mancuso et al	2003	C
	Marks	2008	C
	Montin et al	2007	C
	Naylor et al	2008	C
	Nickinson et al	2009	C
	Ostendorf et al	2004	C
	Parsons et al	2009	C
	Vincent et al	2007	C
	Wang et al	2010	C
	Wang and Emery	2002	C
	Wong et al	2002	C
	Oberg et al	2005	D
	Thomas et al	2010	D
Reduced anxiety	McDonald et al	2014	A
	McDonald et al	2004	A
	Coudeyre et al	2007	B
	Crowe and Henderson	2003	B
	Johansson et al	2007	B

Category	Author	Year	Evidence quality
	Rivard et al	2003	B
	Drummond et al	2012	C
	Fielden et al	2003	C
	Montin et al	2007	C
	Orpen and Harris	2010	C
	Soever et al	2010	C
	Spalding	2004	C
	Spalding	2003	C
	Heine et al	2004	D
	Hunt et al	2009	D
Resumption of meaningful occupation	Malviya et al	2014	A
	Smith et al	2015	B
	Abe et al	2014	C
	Bohm	2010	C
	Cowie et al	2013	C
	Gillen et al	2007	C
	Grant et al	2009	C
	Harding et al	2014	C
	McHugh and Luker	2012	C
	Nunley et al	2011	C
	Ollivier et al	2014	C
	Sankar et al	2013	C
	Vissers et al	2013	C
	Wagenmakers et al	2011	C
	Williams et al	2012	C
	de Groot et al	2008	D
	Heiberg et al	2013	D
	Mobasheri et al	2006	D
	Parsons et al	2009	D
	Wilson and Villar	2011	D
Hip precautions	Smith et al	2016	A
	Barnsley et al	2015	B
	Hol et al	2010	B

Category	Author	Year	Evidence quality
	Peak et al	2005	B
	Restrepo et al	2011	B
	van der Weegen et al	2016	B
	Ververeli et al	2009	B
	Coole et al	2013	C
	Drummond et al	2012	C
	McQuaid et al	2014	C
	Smith and Sackley	2016	C
	Stewart and McMillan	2011	C
	Malik et al	2002	D
	O'Donnell et al	2006	D
Enhanced recovery	Khan et al	2008	A
	Ibrahim et al	2013	B
	Kim et al	2003	B
	Arshad et al	2014	C
	Berend et al	2004	C
	Bottros et al	2010	C
	Brunenberg et al	2005	C
	Husted et al	2008	C
	Iyengar et al	2007	C
	Pape et al	2013	C
	Siggeirsdottir et al	2005	C
	Aasvang et al	2015	D
Reduced demand on support services	Chow	2001	C

Details on specific limitations of individual studies are noted in the evidence tables in Appendix 7.

A limitation of this guideline is that evidence was not available to enable recommendations to be made about the specific contribution of occupational therapy to total hip replacement service user outcomes. This is reflective of the evidence, but also of the nature of the intervention, which has a core surgical focus and which is essentially multidisciplinary.

The guideline development group was aware that there were some expectations, from College Specialist Section members, that this practice guideline would produce occupational therapy-specific recommendations for hip precautions. The nature of the evidence available at the time of the guideline development and review has not enabled this expectation to be fulfilled.

The need for a randomised controlled trial of hip precautions in occupational therapy has, however, been identified as being essential in order to determine whether precautions are effective (Drummond et al 2012).

The involvement of the College and the Specialist Section in the development, authoring and funding of this practice guideline is fully acknowledged (section 10.6). Involvement is inherent because of the organisational structure of the professional body and its relationship with its members.

The potential for any bias in development and authoring was, however, minimised through the rigorous nature of the guideline development process. This was achieved through the systematic methodology adopted, the contributions of stakeholders and patients, the valued opinions of the independent peer reviewers and occupational therapy end users, and the judicious management of any potential or actual conflicts of interest.

13 Updating the guideline

The National Executive Committee of the Royal College of Occupational Therapists Specialist Section – Trauma and Orthopaedics is responsible for monitoring new evidence over the next five-year period and will provide a focal point for feedback received following publication of the 2nd edition of the guideline.

In line with College procedures, this reviewed guideline will be available until 2022; however, a review may be initiated before this time if there is significant new evidence identified which may impact on practice. Details about the updating and review process are set out in the *Practice guideline development manual* (COT 2017a), available at: *www.rcot.co.uk/practice-resources/rcot-practice-guidelines*.

Further information about the Royal College of Occupational Therapists Specialist Section – Trauma and Orthopaedics is available at: *www.rcot.co.uk/about-us/specialist-sections/trauma-and-orthopaedics-rcot-ss*.

Appendix 1: Guideline development and review groups

Guideline Development Group 2010–2012

Lauren Porter BSc Occupational Therapy, Project Lead

- Senior Occupational Therapist, Orthopaedics, Abergele Hospital, Betsi Cadwalader University Health Board
- RCOTSS – Trauma and Orthopaedics: National Executive Committee Wales Representative (Acting Chair 2010 – February 2012)

Christine Gibb DipCOT

- Occupational Therapist/Team Leader, Imperial College Healthcare NHS Trust, London
- RCOTSS – Trauma and Orthopaedics: Member

Sheila Harrison MSc Occupational Therapy, BA, DipCOT

- Senior Occupational Therapist, Trauma and Orthopaedics, Birmingham Heartlands Hospital, Heart of England Foundation Trust
- RCOTSS – Trauma and Orthopaedics: Member

Shirley McCourt BA (Hons) Health and Social Care, BSc Occupational Therapy

- Head Occupational Therapist, Golden Jubilee National Hospital, Scotland
- RCOTSS – Trauma and Orthopaedics: National Executive Committee Scotland and Northern Ireland Representative

Jade Cope BSc Occupational Therapy

- Occupational Therapist Lead – Trauma and Orthopaedics, Guy's and St Thomas' Hospital, London
- RCOTSS – Trauma and Orthopaedics: Chair (February 2012 to November 2013)

Kate Robertson MSc, PGCert (Falls and Osteoporosis), DipCOT

- Consultant Therapist in Falls Prevention, County Health Partnerships, Nottinghamshire
- RCOTSS – Older People: Falls Clinical Forum Lead

Guideline Review Group 2015–2017

Lauren Porter BSc Occupational Therapy, Project Lead

- Senior Occupational Therapist, Orthopaedics, Abergele Hospital, Betsi Cadwalader University Health Board
- RCOTSS – Trauma and Orthopaedics: National Executive Committee Wales Representative

Sheila Harrison MSc Occupational Therapy, BA, DipCOT

- Senior Occupational Therapist, Trauma and Orthopaedics, Good Hope Hospital, Heart of England Foundation Trust
- RCOTSS – Trauma and Orthopaedics: National Executive Committee Northern England Representative

Jamie McNaught

- Clinical Specialist Occupational Therapist, Orthopaedics, Golden Jubilee National Hospital
- RCOTSS – Trauma and Orthopaedics: National Executive Committee Chair (September 2016 to present)

Sally Taylor

- Clinical Lead – Occupational Therapy, Trauma and Orthopaedics, Wirral University Teaching Hospital NHS Foundation Trust
- RCOTSS – Trauma and Orthopaedics: National Executive Committee Chair (November 2013 to September 2016)

Appendix 2: Acknowledgements

The guideline development group would like to thank all those who have contributed to the development and review of the practice guideline.

A2.1 Guideline development (1st edition 2012)

Stakeholder representatives

- Mr John F Nolan MB, BS, FRCS, FRCS (Orth), Consultant Orthopaedics and Trauma Surgeon and Clinical Director, Orthopaedics Department, Norfolk and Norwich University Hospital NHS Foundation Trust. Member, Executive Committee, British Hip Society
- Brian Lucas RGN, PhD, Lead Nurse Practice and Innovation, The Queen Elizabeth Hospital, King's Lynn NHS Trust, Norfolk; Chair RCN Society of Orthopaedics and Trauma Nursing
- Joe Godden, Professional Officer, Adults, British Association of Social Work; Training Co-ordinator Trafford Carers Centre, Manchester
- Janet Thomas, Chair: Chartered Society of Physiotherapy; Chartered Physiotherapists working with older people (AGILE)
- Carolyn Naisby, Chair, Vicky Cattell, London Branch Secretary: Chartered Society of Physiotherapy; Association of Orthopaedics Chartered Physiotherapists (AOCP)
- Royal College of Surgeons (England): Head of Communications – Policy and Communications

Service user reference groups

- Golden Jubilee National Hospital, Scotland service users
- Rushcliffe 50+ Forum Health Sub Group, Nottinghamshire

The Clinical Governance and Risk Management Development Unit (CGRMDU), arthroplasty team and volunteers at the Golden Jubilee National Hospital are acknowledged for their assistance in the service user consultation and support for the project.

Mrs Sue Knowles, Chair of the Rushcliffe 50+ Forum Health Sub Group, is acknowledged for her assistance in facilitation of the consultation with service users and members of the Health Sub Group.

External peer reviewers

- Lisa Stewart, MSc Primary Care, BScOT, Falls Co-ordinator, Edinburgh Community Health Partnership
- Vicki Cattell, MSc, MCSP, Clinical Specialist Physiotherapist Orthopaedics, Guy's and St Thomas' NHS Foundation Trust, London

Co-opted group members

- Dr Elizabeth White PhD, Head of Research and Development, Royal College of Occupational Therapists
- Mandy Sainty MSc, DipCOT, Research and Development Manager, Royal College of Occupational Therapists

Additional thanks

The guideline development group would also like to thank the following:

- Members of the British Association of Occupational Therapists and their colleagues who contributed views and comments on the draft guideline during the consultation period.
- The Royal College of Occupational Therapists' Practice Publications Group and supporting officers Julia Roberts, Quality Programme Manager, and Tessa Fincham, Publications Manager.
- The Royal College of Occupational Therapists' Library Service.

A2.2 Guideline review (2nd edition 2017)

Stakeholder representatives

Four stakeholders responded to the consultation and the following agreed to be acknowledged:

- Andrew J Hamer, Consultant Orthopaedic Surgeon, Sheffield Teaching Hospitals NHS Trust and Honorary Secretary British Hip Society
- Fiona Balance, Team Lead Occupational Therapist, Orthopaedics and Surgical, Greater Glasgow and Clyde NHS

Service user representatives

Service user views were solicited via Arthritis Care (contacts who had hip replacements) and the National Rheumatoid Arthritis Society (via social media contacts and members). No responses were obtained.

External peer reviewers

- Professor Avril Drummond, Occupational Therapist and Professor of Healthcare Research, School of Health Sciences, University of Nottingham
- Dr Toby Smith, Lecturer in Physiotherapy, University of East Anglia

Co-opted group members

- Melanie Leighton, Occupational Therapy Team Leader for Surgery and Orthopaedics, Frimley Health NHS Foundation Trust
- Paul Marshall-Taylor, Acting Principal Occupational Therapist, Trauma and Orthopaedics, St George's University Hospitals NHS Foundation Trust
- Matt Worthy, Clinical Specialist Occupational Therapist: Orthopaedics, Sheffield Teaching Hospitals

Appendix 3: Service user consultation (1st edition – 2012)

A3.1 Service user groups

The consultation process involved two service user groups.

Group 1: Golden Jubilee National Hospital in Scotland service users
The Golden Jubilee National Hospital (GJNH) is the National Waiting Times Centre for Scotland and provides elective hip replacement surgery for service users from across Scotland. Service users undergoing elective total hip replacement at GJNH are clinically reviewed through the arthroplasty service 12 weeks post-surgery and then at yearly intervals.

The Scottish representative on the guideline development group worked with the clinical governance and risk management development unit (CGRMDU) at GJNH to develop a process for service user engagement as part of the development of this guideline. Ethical approval was not deemed necessary as the service user involvement was defined as evaluation/consultation, with all stages of the process monitored through the clinical governance and risk management development unit.

Group 2: Rushcliffe 50+ Forum Health Sub Group
The Rushcliffe 50+ Forum is a group of people aged over 50 who are registered with a general practitioner within the Rushcliffe Principia Clinical Commissioning Group (CCG) locality and who work in partnership with statutory, voluntary and community organisations to develop and improve public services. Rushcliffe borough is the most southerly borough in the county of Nottinghamshire, bordering Lincolnshire and Leicestershire. The Health Sub Group is a sub-committee of the 50+ Forum, which focuses on local health issues.

A guideline development group member worked with the Chair of the Forum to facilitate involvement of the Health Sub Group in the consultation.

A3.2 Consultation process

The aim of the consultation was to seek service user perspectives on the importance of the service user-centred and service delivery-centred outcomes identified within the scope:

- **Reduced anxiety**
  Feeling confident about what was going to happen and how I would manage.
- **Maximised functional independence**
  Being independent with everyday tasks, i.e. getting washed, dressing, making something to eat.
- **Reduced demand on services**
  Not having to rely on services for support with things I can usually do myself.

- **Resumption of roles**
  Getting back to my usual occupations, i.e. employment, housework, caring for others.
- **Reintegration into community**
  Resuming social activities with family and friends.
- **Reduced length of hospital stay**
  Not being in hospital any longer than necessary.
- **Low readmission rates**
  Not needing to go back into hospital because of unexpected problems after going home.

The guideline development group member working with the Chair of the Rushcliffe 50+ Forum arranged to attend a meeting of the Health Sub Group in August 2011. The purpose of this was to explain the total hip replacement guideline development project and to seek opinion on the form to be used in the consultation with service users and the accompanying letter.

The consultation form asked service users to consider the outcome statements identified by the expert practitioners in the guideline development group and rank them in order of importance by putting a number in the column beside each one to indicate which they considered to be the most important (for example, if maximised functional independence was most important to them, put a 1 in the box, if reduced anxiety was least important put 7, etc.).

The guideline development group member was able to consult with the group (23 members were in attendance) regarding the content of the draft letter and consultation form. Members of the group gave feedback and, where possible, comments were incorporated within the final version used in the consultation.

A3.3 Consultation documents

Group 1: Golden Jubilee National Hospital in Scotland service users consultation
All activities were approved by the CGRMDU and carried out with the support of the clinical governance team, arthroplasty service and volunteers at the hospital. The CGRMDU was able to produce a list of service users undergoing total hip replacement during January 2011. A review of the occupational therapy documentation did not identify any concerns about the appropriateness of contacting these individuals. An introductory letter, consultation form and Freepost return envelopes were sent in August 2011 to the first 50 service users on that list. Individuals were given one month in which to respond. A further 50 service users who attended the arthroplasty clinic for their 12-week clinical review appointment were also asked to complete the consultation form during November and December 2011.

Group 2: Rushcliffe 50+ Forum Health Sub Group consultation
Fifty copies of the letter and consultation form were taken to a wider meeting of the 50+ forum in September 2011. The Chair of the Forum identified that there was no need for this process to seek governance approval from the Primary Care Trust as it had been agreed that the consultation information would be left for people to take if they wished and that a Freepost envelope would be provided for any replies.

A3.4 Consultation results

Support was received from the clinical governance and risk management development unit at GJNH to collate and analyse the returned consultation forms (Table A1).

Table A1: Consultation method and response

Method	Issued	Returned	Completed	Partially completed
GJNH Postal	50	28	10	18
GJNH Arthroplasty Clinic	50	50	31	19
Rushcliffe	39	5	3	2
Total	**139**	**83**	**44**	**39**

The responses were grouped (Table A2) to produce three levels of importance:

High = Ranking 1 and 2

Moderate = Ranking 3, 4 and 5

Low = Ranking 6 and 7

Table A2: Service user priorities for outcomes

Outcome	Level of importance		
	High	Moderate	Low
Maximised functional independence	32	11	1
Reduced anxiety	18	14	12
Resumption of roles	14	19	11
Low readmission rates	11	14	19
Decreased length of hospital stay	7	21	16
Reduced demand on support services	5	29	10
Reintegration into community	3	23	18

The overall response rate and number of individual comments suggested service users were keen to share their perspectives of what was important to them following total hip replacement. The consultation demonstrated the high level of importance service users placed on functional independence, reduction of anxiety and the ability to resume their roles. The order of priority for the remaining outcomes, from highest to lowest, was low readmission rates, decreased length of hospital stay, reduced demand on support services and, finally, reintegration into the community.

In addition to the ranking of the outcomes, a number of qualitative comments were received. Many of these related to the overall experience of receiving a hip replacement.

The responses received from individuals involved will have been influenced by their expectations, experiences and personal circumstances and therefore cannot be said to be totally representative of the population of service users who experience occupational therapy in the context of a total hip replacement. Additionally, the sample does not profess to provide a fully culturally representative perspective. Nonetheless, the consultation provided some invaluable insights into the views of the service user group, views which have influenced the development and presentation of this guideline's recommendations.

Appendix 4: Conflicts of interest declarations

Declarations were made in line with the conflict of interest procedures (COT 2017a) during the original development and during the guideline review process as follows:

- Membership of the Royal College of Occupational Therapists Specialist Section – Trauma and Orthopaedics by all members of the core guideline development group and the review group.
- Membership of the Royal College of Occupational Therapists Specialist Section – Older People by one member of the core guideline development group.
- Position as an Officer of the Royal College of Occupational Therapists by the co-opted editorial lead in the 1st and 2nd editions.
- Position as an Officer of the Royal College of Occupational Therapists by the two co-opted critical appraisers in the 1st edition.
- A therapeutic or operational service head relationship between a member of the guideline development group and the service users consulted in Scotland in the 1st edition.
- An external peer reviewer was a co-author of one of the items of evidence in the 1st edition; both external peer reviewers were co-authors of items of evidence used to support recommendations in the 2nd edition.
- External peer reviewers and stakeholders identified their membership of professional organisations.

The nature of declarations, made by all those involved in the guideline development or its review, was related to professional interests and expertise in clinical practice, education or research. There were nil patient conflicts of interest declared other than personal experience of a total hip replacement.

No commercial or financial interests were declared.

The adherence to the Royal College of Occupational Therapists' conflicts of interest policy, and the nature and management of the above declarations, together with the robust guideline development and review methodology, means that the potential for any bias has been taken into account and mitigated.

Appendix 5: Literature search strategy (1st edition – 2012)

Table A3: Search terms and strings

1 **Hip operation and related terms**	2 **ADL and related terms**	3 **Home environment and related terms**	4 **Client engagement and related terms**	5 **Care pathways and related terms**	6 **Multiple pathology and related terms**	7 **Outcomes and related terms**	8 **Occupational therapy and related terms**
1.0 hip surg* OR hip arthroplasty OR hip operation* OR total hip replacement OR hip joint* OR orthopaedic* surgery OR orthopedic* surgery OR elective surgery OR hip resurfacing OR hip re-surfacing OR **NOT** child* OR hemiarthroplasty OR hemi-arthroplasty OR hemi arthroplasty OR	2.0. activities of daily living OR ADL OR functional status OR functional ability OR physical activity OR mobility OR mobilisation OR return adj to work OR role resum* OR resum* adj 3 role carer	3.0 home environment OR safe environment OR home layout OR mobility aids OR mobility transfer OR adaptive equip* OR equip* OR assistive device* OR assistive technolog* OR adapt* adj home OR bathboard OR perch stool OR walking aid OR chair OR bed OR toilet OR bathroom OR stairs OR access* OR aid* to daily living OR	4.0 fear adj patient* OR anxi* adj patient* OR client centred OR client-centred OR client* needs OR client* preference OR client* satisfaction OR client* expectation* OR expert patient* OR patient centred OR patient-centred	5.0 preoperative OR pre operative OR pre-operative OR perioperative OR post operative OR post-operative OR pre op* assessment OR pre op* intervention OR pre op* education OR risk adj reduce* OR patient education 5.1 acute care OR care plan* OR care pathway OR community adj rehabilitation OR discharge adj home OR	6.0 multiple pathology* OR cognitive dysfunction OR dementia OR learning disab* OR depression OR psycho*	7.0 outcome* OR assess* OR rehabilitat*	8.0 Occupational therap* OR Occupational therapist*

1 **Hip operation and related terms**	2 **ADL and related terms**	3 **Home environment and related terms**	4 **Client engagement and related terms**	5 **Care pathways and related terms**	6 **Multiple pathology and related terms**	7 **Outcomes and related terms**	8 **Occupational therapy and related terms**
		step negotiation OR stair negotiation OR		discharge adj plan* OR enhanced recovery OR inpatient rehabilitation OR inpatient therapy OR rapid recovery OR re-ablement OR reablement OR re-enablement OR re enablement OR discharge adj support OR rehabilitat* OR supportive discharge			
1.1 hip precaution OR hip-precaution OR joint protection OR joint adj school OR hip restriction OR hip dislocation OR				5.2 cost* OR cost effect* OR economic* OR benefit OR			

Note: Asterisks were used as a wild card symbol for truncation.

Table A4: Database search strategy

The search strategy combinations were replicated across the six core databases. The numbers of findings per search are detailed in this table.
In each case terms were searched within the title, subject headings and abstract unless there was an indication to apply exceptions or modifications to improve sensitivity and relevance of the search for that particular database. Exceptions are detailed below.

Search no.	Search strings (see columns in Table A3)	CINAHL	Medline	AMED	PsycINFO	Social Policy and Practice	HMIC
S1	1.0 + 2.0	No. of results: 185 1.0 in title 2.0 in title, abstract and keywords	No. of results: 348 1.0 in title 2.0 in title abstract, and keywords	No. of results: 82 1.0 + 2.0 in title, abstract and subject headings	No. of results: 43 1.0 + 2.0 in title, abstract and subject headings	No. of results: 5 1.0 + 2.0 in title, abstract and subject headings	No. of results: 14 1.0 + 2.0 in title, abstract and subject headings
S2	1.0 + 3.0	No. of results: 58 1.0 in title 3.0 in title, abstract and keywords	No. of results: 119 1.0 in title 3.0 in title, abstract and keywords	No. of results: 67 1.0 + 3.0 in title, abstract and subject headings	No. of results: 7 1.0 + 3.0 in title, abstract and subject headings	No. of results: 1 1.0 + 3.0 in title, abstract and subject headings	No. of results: 8 1.0 + 3.0 in title, abstract and subject headings
S3	1.0 + 4.0	No. of results: 14 1.0 in title 4.0 in title, abstract, and keywords	No. of results: 13 1.0 in title 4.0 in title, abstract, and keywords	No. of results: 29 1.0 + 4.0 in title, abstract and keywords	No. of results: 25 1.0 + 4.0 in title, abstract and keywords	No. of results: 1 1.0 + 4.0 in title, abstract and keywords	No. of results: 5 1.0 + 4.0 in title, abstract and keywords
S4	1.0 + 1.1 + 5.0+ 7.0	No. of results: 194 1.0 + 1.1 in title 5.0 + 7.0 in title, abstract and keywords	No. of results: 331 1.0 + 1.1 in title and keyword 5.0 + 7.0 in title, abstract and keywords	No. of results: 107 1.0 + 1.1 + 5.0 in title, abstract and keywords	No. of results: 44 1.0 + 1.1 + 5.0 in title, abstract and keywords	No. of results: 6 1.0 + 1.1 + 5.0 in title, abstract and keywords	No. of results: 25 1.0 + 1.1 + 5.0 in title, abstract and keywords

Search no.	Search strings (see columns in Table A3)	CINAHL	Medline	AMED	PsycINFO	Social Policy and Practice	HMIC
S5	1.0 + 5.1 + 7.0	No. of results: 350 1.0 in title and keywords 5.1 + 7.0 in title, abstract and keywords	No. of results: 450 1.0 in title and keywords 5.1 in title, abstract and keywords 7.0 in title and keywords	No. of results: 211 1.0 + 5.1 in title, abstract and keywords	No. of results: 39 1.0 + 5.1 in title, abstract and keywords	No. of results: 9 1.0 + 5.1 in title, abstract and keywords	No. of results: 21 1.0 + 5.1 in title, abstract and keywords
S5.1	1.0 + 5.1 + 8.0	No. of results: 29 1.0 in title + subject 5.1 + 8.0 in title, abstract and subject					
S6	1.0 + 5.2 + 7.0	No. of results: 100 1.0 in title 5.2 in title and keywords	No. of results: 317 1.0 in title and keywords 5.2 in title and keywords	No. of results: 61 1.0 and 5.2 in title, abstract and keywords	No. of results: 38 1.0 and 5.2 in title, abstract and keywords	No. of results: 1 1.0 and 5.2 in title, abstract and keywords	No. of results: 34 1.0 and 5.2 in title, abstract and keywords
S7	1.0 + 6.0	No of results: 26 1.0 in title, abstract and keywords 6.0 in title and keywords	No. of results: 18 1.0 in title and keywords 6.0 in title and keywords	No. of results: 48 1.0 and 6.0 in title, abstract and keywords	No. of results: 61 1.0 and 6.0 in title, abstract and keywords	No. of results: 2 1.0 and 6.0 in title, abstract and keywords	No. of results: 10 1.0 and 6.0 in title, abstract and keywords

Table A5: Additional and specialist searches

Search description	Search date	Results
Cochrane Library of systematic reviews and clinical trials. String 1.0 and Recover* or rehabilitat* or outcome or activit* or function	19/09/2011	38
OTDBASE. Search terms: "hip replacement" or "hip operation" or "hip arthroplasty"	19/09/2011	10
OT SEARCH. Search terms: "hip replacement" or "hip operation" or "hip arthroplasty"	19/09/2011	19
OTseeker. Search terms: ("hip replacement" or "hip operation" or "hip arthroplasty") AND (recover* or outcome or "Activities of Daily Living" or function or mobility) AND NOT (Child or hemiarthroplasty)	19/09/2011	13
NHS Economic Evaluation Database (NHS EED). Search terms: "hip replacement" or "hip operation" or "hip arthroplasty"	19/09/2011	11

Appendix 6: Literature search strategy (2nd edition – 2017)

Table A6: Search terms and strings

1. Hip terms	2. Generic occupational therapy related terms	3. Occupational therapy	4. Desired outcomes	5. Finance/value terms
Hip N2/adj2* OR Arthroplasty OR Surgical OR Surgery OR Replac* OR Resurfac* OR Re-surfac*OR Operate OR Operated OR Operates OR Operation	Rehabilit* OR Reablement OR Re-ablement OR Re-enable* OR Assessment* OR Educate OR Education OR Expert patient OR Activities of daily living OR ADL OR IADL OR Instrumental activities of daily living OR Function* OR Independen* OR Therapeutic* OR Occupation OR Activit* OR Daily living skills OR Personal care OR Self care OR Self-care OR Participation OR Engage OR Engaged OR Engaging OR Engagement	Occupational therap*	Recover* OR Reduc* N2/adj3 anxiety OR Reduc* N2/adj3 fear OR "Rapid recovery" OR "Enhanced recover" OR "Accelerated discharge" OR Function* N2/adj3 resum* OR Role* N2/adj3 resum* OR "Return to work" OR "Reintergrat* N2/adj3 community" OR Reduc* N2/adj3 readmission* OR Reduc*N2/adj3 re-admission* OR Reduc N2/adj3 hospital stay	Econom* OR Cost* OR Financ* OR Money OR Monies OR Saving* OR Resource* OR Staff*

Note: Asterisks were used as a wild card symbol for truncation.

Table A7: Core platforms and databases

Database or platform and search date	**EBSCO**	**Ovid**
	13/11/15	**16/11/15**
Search term strings (below) and fields searched (right)	ti, ab, su	ti, ab, de, hw, id
Strings: 1 AND 3	39	8
Strings: 1 AND 2 AND 3	28	5
Strings: 1 AND 2 AND 4	430	0
Strings: 1 AND 3 AND 5	10	2
Strings: 1 AND 2 AND 3 AND 5	7	2
Strings: 1 AND 2 AND 4 AND 5	31	0
Total results	545	17
Removed via platform de-duping and/or filter options	*80*	*9*
Total for cleansing within and across databases	**465**	**8**

Medline, CINAHL – accessed via EBSCOHOST platform
AMED, HMIC, PsycINFO, Social Policy and Practice – accessed via OVID platform

Table A8: Specialist databases

Database or platform	**Fields**	**Terms**	**Number transferred**	**Date of search**
Cochrane	ti, ab, kw	1 Hip surg* or hip arthroplasty or hip operation or total hip replacement or hip joint or hip resurfacing or hip re-surfacing or Orthopaedics surgery or Orthopaedics 2 Recover* or rehabilitat* or outcome or activit* or function 3 Occupational therap* 4 Economic or cost or finance or money or monies or saving* or resource or staff String 1 AND 2 String 1 AND 3 String 1 AND 2 AND 4	**78**	20/11/15
OT Search	All fields	"Hip replacement" or "hip operation" or "hip arthroplasty"	**6**	23/11/15

Database or platform	Fields	Terms	Number transferred	Date of search
OTseeker	ti, ab	1 Hip replacement or hip operation or hip arthroplasty 2 Hip replacement or hip operation or hip arthroplasty AND recover* or outcome or Activities of Daily Living or function or mobility	**16**	23/11/15
OTDBASE	Topic search ti, ab	"Hip replacement" or "hip operation" or "hip arthroplasty"	**2**	20/11/15
NICE/SIGN	Hand search	"Hip replacement" or "hip operation" or "hip arthroplasty"	**30**	25/11/15
RCOT Library	All fields	"Hip replacement" or "hip operation" or "hip arthroplasty"	**0**	25/11/15

Key:

ab = abstract	de = descriptors	hw = heading words	id = key words
kw = keyword	sh = subject heading	su = subject	ti = title

Appendix 7: Evidence tables

Source	Design and participants	Intervention	Outcome measures	Results	Quality and comment
Aasvang et al (2015)	Narrative review of literature by anaesthetists Aim: to review outcomes following fast-track/enhanced recovery programmes Denmark.	Total hip and knee arthroplasty.	• Ongoing pain up to 2 weeks post-operatively • Stress post-operatively • Function post-op • Lower limb muscle loss and engagement in physiotherapy • Delirium and cognitive problems post-operatively • Sleep disturbance • Increased anxiety and low self-esteem due to pain.	Whilst people may leave hospital quicker due to fast-track programmes, they will still encounter significant challenges post-operatively (pain, sleep, delirium and cognitive function) Authors conclude that future focus should not only be on further length of stay (LOS) reduction but on identifying and reducing the decline in post-discharge physical and cognitive function, and the surgical/medical complications in high-risk patients.	Grade D – Very Low Comments: • Small narrative review • Focus from anaesthetics.
Abe et al (2014)	Cohort study Aim: to understand if individuals jog post-total hip replacement (THR) surgery and if not, why not Recruitment between 2005–2011 via 2 hospitals Inclusion: underwent primary THR 608 participants 527 THR 81 hip resurfacing Mean age = 62 years Male:female ratio = 85:523 Japan.	Total hip arthroplasty.	• X-rays • Service user activity questionnaires, including questions about jogging • Western Ontario and McMaster Universities Osteoarthritis Index (WOMAC) and University of California, Los Angeles (UCLA) activity scales administered • Serial radiographs performed to measure any implant loosening, bearing wear or osteolysis around the components.	• 33 participants jogged pre-operatively and 23 post-operatively. Of these, 10 had hip resurfacing surgery • 3.8% of participants jogged post-THR and follow-up revealed no negative effect on the implant from jogging • 87% of participants said they had no interest in jogging • Of 74 participants who had interest in jogging but weren't, 45 said because of anxiety, 18 said impossible because of pain, decreased range of movement and muscle weakness, and 11 patients said because of lumbar or knee pain.	Grade C – Low Comments: • Disproportionate ratio of women to men, so cannot generalise results to all • Only looked at the effect on the prosthesis of the joggers • A range of hip implants were used – not possible to differentiate • Follow-up only up to 4.8 years.

Source	Design and participants	Intervention	Outcome measures	Results	Quality and comment
Alviar et al (2011)	Review of evidence Aim: to compare eight patient-reported outcome measures used in hip and knee arthroplasty to the International Classification of Functioning, Disability and Health (ICF) Inclusion: patient-reported, multi-dimensional outcome measures in prospective studies and reviews involving arthroplasty patients undergoing any rehabilitation intervention/discipline ('multi-dimensional' defined as two or more domains with at least one on activity or participation); studies with the aim of examining any of the measurement properties of the instruments Exclusion: non-English studies, theses, conference proceedings and studies with a sample size of <10 68 studies examining 23 instruments, though eight instruments formed the basis of the review.	Hip and knee arthroplasty Outcome measures focused on function, activity and participation The contents of each measure were linked to the ICF based on established ICF linking rules. The item was extracted from the patient-reported outcome measure and then the meaningful concepts per items were identified. These meaningful concepts were then linked to the most specific ICF category.	Instruments included: • Western Ontario and McMaster Universities Osteoarthritis Index • Oxford Knee Score • Oxford Hip Score • Knee Injury and Osteoarthritis Outcome Score • Hip Dysfunction and Osteoarthritis Outcome Score • Lequesne Algofunctional Index • Health Assessment Questionnaire • Arthritis Impact Measurement Scales.	• 229 (61%) concepts were able to be mapped to the activity and participation component of the ICF • Not all relevant activity and participation issues were fully captured by any of the tools • Significant environmental factors were not addressed in the majority of tools • These instruments have some gaps in coverage for significant areas of activity, participation and environment that are necessary in adequately assessing rehabilitation outcomes. This could be a limitation when used in arthroplasty rehabilitation outcome studies, but also provides the basis for further development of outcome assessment instruments.	Grade B – Moderate Downgraded due to: • Not a systematic review • Could increase number of raters reviewing the assessments and ICF criteria • The ICF core set was specific to osteoarthritis, not exclusive to hips and knees • Personal factors not included in ICF – need to probe more psychometric attributes.

Source	Design and participants	Intervention	Outcome measures	Results	Quality and comment
Arshad et al (2014)	Matched cohort study Aim: to assess the effectiveness of the Norwich Enhanced Recovery Programme versus a non-enhanced recovery programme following total hip replacement (THR) and total knee replacement (TKR) (evidence table focuses solely on THR) Inclusion: primary THR Enhanced recovery group n=48 Male:female ratio = 23:25 Standard pathway group n=48 Male:female ratio = 14:34 Similar characteristics in both except gender United Kingdom.	• Multi-modal analgesia • Pre-operative education • Early mobilisation.	Primary outcome was hospital length of stay Secondary outcomes: • Post-operative complications and need for further surgery within 6 weeks • Post-operative haemoglobin • Post-operative blood transfusion • Discharge destination • Discharge walking aid.	• Reduced length of stay in enhanced recovery group – not statistically significant • Statistically significant levels of haemoglobin in enhanced recovery group • Statistically significant difference in participants discharged straight home (not to rehabilitation): enhanced recovery 96%, standard pathway 65% ($p<0.01$).	Grade C – Low Comments: • Larger number of females in standard pathway group.

Source	Design and participants	Intervention	Outcome measures	Results	Quality and comment
Barnsley et al (2015)	Systematic review Aim: to review the evidence on whether hip precautions versus unrestricted activities significantly decrease the risk of prosthetic dislocation Inclusion: RCT or cohort studies with comparison group, at least 6 months' follow-up and have specific information on hip dislocation and re-operation, English language articles only from 2000 onwards Exclusion: case series and case reports 2 studies included = 346 patients Studies: Peak et al 2005; Ververeli et al 2009.	Hip precautions.	Dislocation post-total hip replacement (THR).	Use of hip precautions in the anterolateral approach does not improve dislocation rates Hip precautions are associated with: • A slower return to activities • Increased expense • Decreased service user satisfaction.	Grade B – Moderate Downgraded due to: • Unfortunate low number of studies due to lack of published research • Lack of detailed data and inability to pool results • Some methodological flaws within included studies affecting quality. Comments: • Only includes articles relating to anterolateral approach.
Berend et al (2004)	Retrospective study Aim: to examine outcomes for a study group who have undergone an enhanced recovery programme compared to a control group No details regarding recruitment or population characteristics Convenience sample comparing pre-programme (168 in the control group) and post-programme (128 in the study group) United States of America.	Enhanced recovery programme for total hip replacement Details poor but programme appeared to include multimodal approach with pre-operative and post-operative education and 'early and aggressive rehabilitation'.	Length of stay (LOS) and readmission rates Discharge location.	• No statistically significant differences noted between groups for height, weight or age ($p>0.05$) • Length of stay was reduced significantly in the study group from 4.04 days in 1997 (range 2–9 days, SD 1.1 days) to 2.66 days in 2003 (range 1–7 days, SD 0.86, $p<0.0001$) • Rate of readmission to hospital within 3 months was significantly lower in the study group (3.9% compared to 8.3%, $p=0.05$). Suggests holistic, peri-operative enhanced recovery programme can reduce length of stay and lower hospital readmission rates.	Grade C – Low Limitations: • Poor information – mostly descriptive/bordering on audit • Retrospective sample with 6-year period between data for control group compared to the study group • May have confounding variables during 6-year period that may have also impacted on results, not just the introduction of the enhanced recovery programme • No power calculation.

Source	Design and participants	Intervention	Outcome measures	Results	Quality and comment
Berge et al (2004)	Randomised controlled trial Aims: 1. Determine effects of Pain Management Programme (PMP) pre-operatively on pain and function while on wait list for total hip replacement (THR) 2. Determine if gains from the PMP allowed patients to decide to delay surgery 3. Measure effects if any on PMP post-operatively PMP group n=19 Mean age 71.6 years Male:female ratio = 7:12 Control group n=21 Mean age 71 years Male:female ratio = 6:15 United Kingdom.	Total hip replacement Treatment group: • Pain management programme • 6 weeks • 2 mornings a week • Total 21 hours input. Control group: • No intervention.	Assessment focus on pain, disability and quality of life through tools: • Pain • Arthritis Impact Measurement Scale (pre- and post-operatively) • Mobility (timed walk) • Sleep • Analgesia consumption • Delays to surgery due to improved condition.	At pre-operative follow-up: 1. Treatment group decrease in average pain intensity, pain distress and pain-related sleep disturbance – statistical significance p=0.003 to p=0.005. No statistical significance with pain relief, Arthritis Impact Measurement Scale (AIMS) total, mobility, depression or physical activity 2. Nil difference between groups in decision to delay surgery 3. 1-year post-operative follow-up the treatment group had statistically significant results (p=0.02) scoring better in AIMS score (physical activity); however, no significant differences in other variables.	Grade B – Moderate Downgraded from Grade A due to limitations: • Small numbers • Drop-outs/exclusions not clear • Small numbers in final analysis: 18 treatment and 15 control • Reasons for exclusions not stated • No information re blinding in the randomisation • No measurement of co-morbid problems which might affect function outcomes.

Source	Design and participants	Intervention	Outcome measures	Results	Quality and comment
Bohm (2010)	Prospective cohort study Aim: to investigate the impact of total hip replacement on a service user's work ability 84 service users on waiting list who were in work pre-operatively (working age only) Response rate 54/60 at the 1-year follow-up. Not all data provided by respondents Return to work group: Mean age 49.9 years Male:female ratio = 21:19 Not returning to work group: Mean age 60.3 years Male:female ratio = 1:5 Canada.	Total hip replacement.	Self-administered questionnaire emailed to participants at 12 months post-operatively Measures varied and included employment status aspects, physical function, hip function, job motivation and satisfaction, workplace demands and flexibility and productivity.	• 38 out of 44 service users who were working pre-operatively had returned to work 1 year post-operatively (86%) • Only one service user attributed stopping work to the hip condition (2%) • 34 out of the 38 service users who returned to work returned to doing the same job • 2 of the 10 service users who were off work pre-operatively had returned to work 1 year post-operatively (20%). Those who were working pre-operatively returned to work at a much higher rate than those not working pre-operatively (p<0.001). Those who returned to work reported better Oxford-12 hip scores, better general physical function scores and fewer limitations from medical conditions.	Grade C – Low Limitations: • No details of how sample selected • Possible volunteer and self-reporting bias • Other factors may have influenced the service user's ability to return to work, such as co-morbidities • Small sample size – no multivariate regression analysis to investigate the individual effects of each variable.
Bottros et al (2010)	Retrospective cohort study Aim: analysis of how implementing an enhanced recovery programme affects length of stay and early post-operative pain control and function 103 service users who had a total hip replacement Enhanced recovery n=30 Traditional programme n=73 Average age 59 years Male:female = 53%:47% United States of America.	Total hip replacement Enhanced recovery: combines surgical approach, protocols focusing on early safe mobilisation of service user and anticipated discharge home on day two or three Traditional approach: bed restriction on day of surgery and anticipated discharge to rehabilitation or home on day four.	Collected on each post-operative day: • Visual analogue scale for pain • Walking distance. Length of stay (LOS) and discharge destination (home or rehabilitation facility) Harris Hip Score collected at 4- and 12-week post-operative visits.	Service users treated with the enhanced recovery programme had: • A decreased average LOS 3.5 days average compared with 4.47 average in traditional group (p=0.02) • Improved walking distance (p=0.01) • Achieved longer walking distances earlier (p<0.05) • Lower visual analogue scale for pain ratings on the 2nd post-operative day (p=0.01) • Trends towards improved Harris Hip Scores also observed in the enhanced recovery group (not statistically significant).	Grade C – Low Limitations: • Did not assess complications and readmissions • Cannot attribute these improvements to any single factor as did not examine the enhanced recovery components individually • Absence of long-term data.

Source	Design and participants	Intervention	Outcome measures	Results	Quality and comment
Brunenberg et al (2005)	Case control study – before and after trial Aim: to examine the cost-effectiveness of a joint recovery programme (JRP) for service users undergoing joint replacement compared to usual care Consecutive recruitment THR and total knee replacement THR group n=98: Mean age 64.4 years JRP n=48 Male:female ratio = 35.4%:64.6% Controls n=50 Male:female ratio = 24%:76% Netherlands.	Total hip or knee replacement Joint recovery programme: • Pre-operative screening and assessment of home/care needs • Information and education (40-minute session, 1–2 weeks pre-operatively) • Group rehabilitation. Control usual care: • No pre-operative screening or education • Conventional physical therapy.	Cost-effectiveness of the joint recovery programme: • Joint improvement • Functional improvement via Harris Hip Score • Quality of life via EQ-5D™ • Hospital length of stay. Costs: pre-admission, admission and post-discharge (up to 1 year post-operatively).	In relation to THR: • Mean joint improvement at 1 year was significantly higher in the JRP group (difference $p=0.035$) • Course of improvement in joint function statistically significantly different between groups ($p=0.012$) • The reduction in hospital length of stay was statistically significant ($p<0.001$) • Quality of life measures were in favour of the intervention group but not statistically significant • Statistically significant in the areas of joint and functional improvement and length of stay • Standardised JRP results in shorter length of stay, better function and less non-attendance for surgery and is therefore cost-effective.	Grade C – Low Limitations: • Small sample size from a single hospital (10 drop-outs) • Deemed unfeasible for randomised controlled trial due to high risk of contamination of data • Single-site study • No reference is made to the potential effect of any individual component of the programme or changes in the physiotherapy programme that resulted in an increased intensity of rehabilitation.
Caracciolo and Giaquinto (2005)	Prospective cohort study Aim: to determine whether psychological distress and depression are associated with reduced functional improvement following joint replacement 36 service users with THR and 36 service users with TKR THR group: Mean age 67.9 years Male:female ratio = 7:29 Rehabilitation facility Italy.	Total hip replacement or total knee replacement.	Administered on admission (baseline) and on discharge (follow-up) • Western Ontario and McMaster Universities Osteoarthritis Index (WOMAC) • The Hospital Anxiety and Depression (HAD) scale.	Results for THR: • 44% of THR service users showed over-threshold HAD scores on admission • Proportion even higher when the HAD Depression subscale examined, 55% of THR service users scoring over-threshold • No difference found between THR depressed versus non-depressed service users on WOMAC gain scores on follow-up • No association found between psychological distress and depression and functional recovery in this group.	Grade C – Low Limitations: • Possible confounding variable of time between surgery and admission to rehabilitation unit which could have impacted function/psychological state • Length of follow-up not adequate to observe effect • No information re referral criteria or if service users consecutively enrolled.

Source	Design and participants	Intervention	Outcome measures	Results	Quality and comment
Chow (2001)	Prospective cohort study Aim: to investigate whether carers experienced stress from looking after individuals with osteoarthritis who were waiting for a THR Convenience sampling 72 participants – initial response rate of 58% gave 34 pairs of caregivers/receivers; 23 out of the 34 pairs participated in second stage Carers: mean age 63 years Male:female ratio = 10:13 Care receivers: Mean age 70 years Male:female ratio = 8:15 United Kingdom.	Total hip replacement.	Completed prior to and 3 months following the hip replacement Service user outcomes: • The Nottingham Health Profile (NHP) • Visual Analogue Pain Scale. Caregiver outcomes: • Robinson's Caregiver Stress Index • Visual Analogue Pain Scale (completed with level of pain caregiver perceived the care receiver to be in).	Care receivers: • NHP – 52.6% significant improvement in mean score post-operatively (p<0.001) • 82.4% reduction in pain intensity score (p<0.001). Carers: • 23% reduction in mean stress score post-operative, but not significant (p<0.06) • Correlation between the health profile of care receivers and carer's stress level pre-operatively high (r=0.82, p<0.05), but almost no relationship 3 months post-THR (r=0.1) • Intensity of pain that the caregiver perceived the care receiver to be in reduced by 65.5% at 3-month post-operative mark (p<0.0001).	Grade C – Low Limitations: • Sample size was small • Data was only collected for a 3-month period post-operatively which is too short to measure outcome • Possible reporter bias as volunteers • Confounding factors (pre-existing co-morbidities or complications that arose from surgery) • There is no evidence of calculation of confidence intervals in this study.

Source	Design and participants	Intervention	Outcome measures	Results	Quality and comment
Coole et al (2013)	Qualitative – semi-structured telephone interviews Aim: to report the views and experiences of clinicians on the use of hip precautions (to reduce the risk of dislocation following total hip replacement) Recruitment via 6 NHS trusts in 6 different regions of England identified by the study's steering committee, with snowballing used once the first participant was recruited 16 healthcare staff Occupational therapists – 6 Orthopaedic surgeons – 4 Physiotherapists – 3 Nurses – 3 United Kingdom.	Total hip replacement precautions.	Themes investigated: • Routine application of hip precautions – rationale, disadvantages and consistency of application • Relaxation of hip precautions – barriers, facilitators, process and impact • Contextual factors – services undergoing change and support for further research.	Variation in views due to difference in surgical opinion and lack of evidence Relaxing routine provision is viewed as having an impact on patient recovery and satisfaction, the role and skill mix of therapy services, and length of hospital stay and resource use More research needed into the effect of hip precautions – especially since little is known about long-term effect on functional activity.	Grade C – Low Comments: • Unable to interview clinicians from each of the professions identified at each site • Unlikely that data saturation reached (small sample, and unlikely to have reflected all the different ways in which hip precautions are applied in the UK) • Interviews conducted by telephone rather than face to face (however, telephone interviews can create greater opportunity for disclosure, and no evidence that data collected of lower quality) • Potential risk of bias as it was not clear how the researchers chose the hospital trusts in the study.

Source	Design and participants	Intervention	Outcome measures	Results	Quality and comment
Coudeyre et al (2007)	Systematic literature review Aim: development of clinical practice guidelines for pre-operative rehabilitation for total hip and knee joint replacement • Systematic literature review • Collection of everyday clinical practice • External review by multidisciplinary team expert panel. 10 studies (9 were randomised controlled trials). Quality assessed – French Agency for Accreditation and Evaluation in Healthcare.	Rehabilitation pre-operatively for total hip or knee joint replacement Interventions were heterogeneous regarding healthcare professional involved, intervention duration and modality Occupational therapy was delivered at home or in hospital. Usually practical, evaluating material and human environment, counselling or advice Some intervention multidisciplinary.	Outcomes considered: • Impairment – restricted range of movement or muscular strength • Disability as measured by validated questionnaire, gait analysis, discharge criteria • Medico-economic implications for length of stay, discharge destination and cost of peri-operative care • Post-operative complications.	Overall results relevant to THR: • Pre-operative rehabilitation has benefit in terms of length of the stay in hospital and destination at discharge • A programme comprising at least physical therapy and education is recommended • Prior to THR occupational therapy should be proposed • Multidisciplinary rehabilitation, comprising occupational therapy and education, is desirable for those service users with major disability, co-morbidity or social problems • Pre-operative evaluation of service user's needs important and advise use of predictive tool such as Risk Assessment and Prediction Tool.	Grade B – Moderate Downgraded from Grade A due to limitations: • Not all studies RCTs and mixed approach • Difficulty isolating the impact of pre-operative rehabilitation from global care consisting of pre- and post-operative rehabilitation • Lack of analysis of post-operative complications as an outcome measure • No written evidence of external review by multidisciplinary team experts.
Cowie et al (2013)	Cohort study Aim: to understand levels of sporting activity and when individuals returned to work post-total hip arthroplasty (THA) Recruitment via one hospital Inclusion: underwent THA 2005–2009 and under age 65 years Total of 285 THAs performed on 239 service users United Kingdom.	Total hip arthroplasty.	• Sporting activity (pre- and post-operatively) • When resumed sports • When returned to work.	• Of 239 service users, 170 working at time of follow-up, 18.6% in heavy manual jobs • On average, it took 13.9 weeks to return to work • It took 18.8 weeks, on average, to return to sport • Those with lower body mass index (BMI) returned to work and sports earlier than those with a higher BMI.	Grade C – Low Comments: • Reinforces existing evidence on THA recovery and experience • Only one hospital, so results may be regionally specific • Co-morbidities not discussed • Baseline of pre-operative activity not evidenced.

Source	Design and participants	Intervention	Outcome measures	Results	Quality and comment
Crowe and Henderson (2003)	Randomised controlled trial (RCT) Aim: what is the effect on length of stay of individually tailored pre-operative rehabilitation for clients with more complex needs undergoing hip or knee replacement? 133 subjects with complex needs receiving elective hip or knee replacement Rehabilitation group n=65 Mean age 66.9 years Male:female ratio = 14:51 Usual care group = 68 Mean age 70.7 years Male:female ratio = 13:55 Canada.	Total hip or knee replacement – random allocation to: • Usual care group: standard pre-operative clinic visit 1–2 weeks prior to surgery • Rehabilitation group: individualised and multidisciplinary • Counselling/ education • Occupational therapy: environmental preparation, education, strategies to improve pre-operative functioning, energy consideration and task simplification. Some received a home visit.	Pre-operative baseline measures: • Oxford Hip Score • Spielberger State Anxiety Inventory (state component). Post-operatively: • Number of days to meeting discharge criteria • Actual length of stay • Discharge destination • Post-operative complications.	Rehabilitation intervention group less anxious before surgery and better prepared in advance for return home • Average number of days to achieve discharge criteria was significantly shorter among pre-operative rehabilitation group (p=0.021) • Length of stay was significantly shorter on average among service users receiving rehabilitation (p=0.032) • Average number of days to meet each individual discharge criterion lower, but most not statistically significant • Significant difference seen in the mean number of days required to have made plans for discharge (equipment, arranged provision of meals), with most in the rehabilitation group having made arrangements prior to admission (p<0.000).	Grade B – Moderate Downgraded from Grade A due to limitations: • Significant differences between groups • No power calculation • Could have more follow-up data • Incompleteness of follow-up in discharge destination • Some difference in type of information or support given pre-operatively • Not all received re-assessment of anxiety • Blind status not possible to achieve but person collating scores blind to the allocation.
de Groot et al (2008)	Cohort study Aim: to assess the effect of THA/TKA on physical activity via use of an activity monitor Long-standing osteoarthritis Excluded co-morbidities 80 (36 THA) service users from pre-assessment to 6 months post-surgery Mean age 61.8 years Male:female ratio = 33:47 Netherlands.	Total hip or knee replacement.	Assessed before surgery, at 3 and 6 months post-operatively • Activity Monitor • WOMAC pain, stiffness and physical function subscales • 6-minute walk test • Chair rising/stair walking • Physical Activities Scale for Individuals with Physical Disability • SF-36® function subscale • Harris Hip Score.	• 0.7% improvement in actual physical activity (p=0.03) – the effect of this was smaller than had been anticipated for 6 months • One THA service user not accounted for at 6 months. Felt by researchers to be too short to show relevant changes in actual activity levels • Self-reported activity increased by 86% – discrepancy between self-report and measured activity • Body function, capacity and self-reported physical functioning improved. Larger effect on pain and stiffness.	Grade D – Very Low Downgraded from Grade C due to limitations: • Likely to be underpowered • Body mass index may be a confounding factor • Sample size small and excluded over 80 years • Follow-up of 6 months too short for general application • Self-reported outcomes may be less reliable than standardised measures • Results combined for THA and TKA groups.

Source	Design and participants	Intervention	Outcome measures	Results	Quality and comment
Drummond et al (2013)	Descriptive analysis Aim: to analyse and evaluate the literature provided to service users by occupational therapists concerning elective hip surgery in the UK Questionnaires posted to occupational therapists requesting copies of information leaflets and booklets given to service users 111 information leaflets and booklets examined United Kingdom.	Service user information literature.	Checklist devised by researchers as evaluation tool to consider: • Accessibility including presentation of information • Breadth of information covered (unclear if solely occupational therapy or wider remit) • Specific activities of daily living described.	• Variation in the readability of leaflets ranging from 13% to 83% (mean 45%, SD 15) • Variation in content ranging from surgery and possible complications to diet and hip exercises • The most commonly covered activity of daily living related to sitting (99, 89%), the least covered was work (26, 23%) • Only 3 (2.7%) involved service users in their production and only 22 (20%) signposted obtaining information in another language or Braille.	Grade C – Low Comments: • Evaluation instrument had to be devised by authors because no suitable tool (which would have been preferable). Instrument's psychometric properties not tested, and recognised as a limitation • The quality of advice given was not evaluated; instead concentrated on whether or not a topic was discussed (thus high score may have been given to a leaflet which had inappropriate advice) • Some limitations regarding scope of literature examined, as some leaflets intended to be used in conjunction with other leaflets. However, study evaluated leaflets individually • No clarity regarding what stage of clinical pathway leaflets were intended to be issued • Recognition that leaflets are an adjunct to therapy and should not be evaluated out of context.

Source	Design and participants	Intervention	Outcome measures	Results	Quality and comment
Drummond et al (2012)	National postal survey Aim: what is routine practice in UK occupational therapy in advising on hip precautions following primary THR? Recruitment: advertising at conferences, COT Specialist Sections, personal contacts and 233 UK NHS hospitals n=236 Postal survey using questionnaire designed by authors and based on literature and expert opinion piloted prior to main survey United Kingdom.	Hip precautions post elective total hip replacement.	• Approximate proportion of caseload THR treated and therapy hours/per service user • Movements service users told to avoid • Activities discussed and practised • When and why precautions taught • Provision of equipment/ home visits and follow-up • Estimated effect of precautions on length of stay • Length of time precautions applied • Use of protocols and service user information.	Response rate of 72% – 174 suitable for analysis (66%) • Generally national agreement on movements service users asked to avoid: flexion, adduction and internal/external rotation • Common activities discussed kitchen activities, bath/shower transfers, car transfers, strip-washing/dressing techniques • Common practised: bed, chair and toilet transfers and dressing • Service users seen pre-surgery from over 8 weeks to 1 week • Reasons for precautions – most popular surgical opinion (72.4%) • Most common equipment prescribed: raised toilet seat (94.8%) • Majority of services did not routinely carry out home visits • Precautions observed range from 6 weeks to over 12 weeks.	Grade C – Low Limitations: • Responses dependent on interest – may not be complete response • The questionnaire not included – difficult to appraise objectivity of questions • Excluded private hospitals – shorter waiting times and access to a range of providers may make rationale for not including less viable • Did not appear to take into account those services with no precautions.

Source	Design and participants	Intervention	Outcome measures	Results	Quality and comment
Fielden et al (2003)	Qualitative study Aim: to investigate service user expectations of and satisfaction with in-hospital discharge planning after THR in early and late discharge service user groups Purposive sample: 33 (over 18 years) recruited during visit to pre-assessment clinic 19 in early discharge group and 14 in late group Two metropolitan hospitals New Zealand.	Total hip replacement Early discharge group – fewer than 5 days in hospital Late discharge group – 5 or more days in hospital.	In-depth semi-structured interview 30 minutes on day of discharge and again 4–8 weeks later either in hospital at follow-up or in their homes Open-ended questions focused on outcome aspects, allowed for service user individual report of experiences.	• No clear difference between two groups. Themes categorised into readying self, recovering mobility and transition to wellness • Written information at pre-assessment appreciated, however reports that there is little if any time for individualised question relevant to their specific concerns • Lack of clarity about discharge planning and roles of multidisciplinary team • Value of equipment to recovery highlighted • Concerns re being told different things by multidisciplinary team members resulting in confusion and difficulty planning for recovery, e.g. when can they drive.	Grade C – Low Limitations: • Only two hospitals sampled – can't generalise • Minimal information on sample characteristics.

Source	Design and participants	Intervention	Outcome measures	Results	Quality and comment
Gillen et al (2007)	Cohort study Aim: to examine effect of occupational therapy intervention focused on improving community skills after a lower extremity major joint replacement (hip and knee replacement) Recruitment: n=107 THR n=32 TKR n=72 Mean age 63.7 years Male:female ratio = 33.6%:66.4% Private rehabilitation centre United States of America.	Total hip or knee replacement Occupational therapy – community reintegration programme – range of external activities Five pre-determined goals: • Entering and exiting a vehicle • Shopping • Managing outdoor obstacles • Participating safely in the community • Travelling to and from outpatient appointments. One session of 45 minutes.	Pre- and post-intervention Adapted version of Canadian Occupational Performance Measure (COPM©) used pre- and post-test Client rates functional abilities in activities of daily living, rating level of performance and satisfaction with performance Confidence scale researcher devised.	Following practice of community skills in a natural environment, satisfaction with performance, and performance of community skills – rated higher ($p<0.0001$) Confidence also higher. Some individuals did report decrease in perceived performance COPM© provides valid and reliable method to evaluate community functioning based upon self-report To optimise rehabilitation outcomes, should focus on enhancing community participation and decreasing activity limitations.	Grade C – Low Limitations: • No details provided on recruitment process which was from one institution and all elective surgery • Self-reported measures only • Confidence measure not validated • No control group for comparison • Need longitudinal follow-up.
Grant et al (2009)	Qualitative study – grounded theory approach Aim: to investigate the processes of recovery from total hip replacement from service user perspective Purposive sampling n=10 Age range 65–84 years Male:female ratio = 4:6 Total hip replacement in previous 4–6 months Regional hospital Australia.	Total hip replacement.	In-depth interviews Interview guide focused on topics related to recovery.	Recovery process – three key themes emerged as interrelating processes within the recovery experience: • Reclaiming physical ability (pacing self, using mobility aids, accepting assistance, maintaining an awareness of risk of injury) • Re-establishing roles and relationships and • Refocusing self. Intervening conditions affecting recovery process include co-morbid conditions, the personal outlook of the service user, service user's relationships and social support.	Grade C – Low Limitations: • Unclear re any bias from research and participant relationship • Processes and structures related to THR surgery may be contextual • All participants returned home after surgery (while some of THR population, as a whole, requires continuing care).

Source	Design and participants	Intervention	Outcome measures	Results	Quality and comment
Harding et al (2014)	Cohort study Aim: to use an accelerometer to measure changes in physical activity in people undergoing THA or TKA from pre-operatively to 6 months post-operatively and determine the proportion of people meeting the American Physical Activity Guidelines Recruitment via large public hospital Inclusion: aged 50–80 with a diagnosis of hip or knee OA, waitlisted for a primary THA or TKA Exclusion: 'wheelchair bound', or living in high-level care facilities, co-morbidities that significantly affected their level of physical activity such as a previous stroke, or those with English language or cognitive barriers 57 participants, 44 with validated data sets THA = 19 participants TKA = 25 participants Mean age = 69 Male:female ratio = 36:64 Australia.	• THA or TKA – types of prosthesis used were dependent on consultant, with options described • Rehabilitation followed same post-operative protocol for all (this was described) and all were weight-bearing as tolerated.	The primary outcome was physical activity, measured via an accelerometer (activity monitor) which was to be worn for a minimum of 10 hours a day (during waking hours) over 7 consecutive days Participants were also given an activity diary to record times when and why the monitor was not worn Secondary outcomes measured were self-reported pain, function, quality of life and physical activity Data collected via: • Oxford Hip and Knee Score • SF-12 Generic Health Survey • UCLA Activity Score • Global Rating of Change (GRC) score for measuring self-perceived change in physical activity.	• There was no change in objectively measured physical activity over time • Pre-operatively, participants spent 82% of the time measured engaged in sedentary activities, compared to 83% at 6 months post-operatively ($p=0.11$) • Very few participants met the American Physical Activity Guidelines either before or after recovery from arthroplasty • Significant improvements in self-reported pain during activity ($p<0.001$), physical function ($p<0.001$), quality of life ($p<0.001$) and in physical activity measured by the UCLA activity score ($p<0.001$).	Grade C – Low Comments: • Small sample size, with perhaps unnecessary loss of participants due to technical problems • Strict exclusion criteria • Short follow-up period • Grouped hip and knee arthroplasties together • Focused on physical activity • Minimal detail on functional improvements post-operatively.

Source	Design and participants	Intervention	Outcome measures	Results	Quality and comment
Heiberg et al (2013)	Cohort study Aim: to describe the desires of a group of service users regarding improvements in physical functioning Recruitment via 2 hospitals between October 2008 and March 2010 Inclusion: diagnosis of primary hip osteoarthritis and residence close to the hospital Exclusion: osteoarthritis of the knee or contralateral hip which restricted walking, a neurological disease, dementia, heart disease, drug abuse and an inadequate ability to read and understand Norwegian 64 participants at 12 months post-operatively Mean age = 65 years Male:female ratio = 30:34 Norway.	Total hip arthroplasty.	Assessing trends in functional goals over a year Participants were asked to describe their functional goals pre-operatively then 3 and 12 months post-operatively Responses coded in line with ICF classification.	• Functional targets decreased as the year progressed • Participants were focused on mobility and independent function • In the first 3 months, the focus was on personal care tasks, e.g. dressing lower body • Post 3 months, the focus was on recreation and leisure, walking and moving around.	Grade D – Very Low Downgraded due to: • No information about surgery or surgical outcomes which may have affected results • Possibility of coding bias • Large number of participants lost at 3-month point – from 128 cohort available, only have full data for 64 which affects generalisability • Cohort not necessarily representative of population, again affecting generalisability. Comments: • Possibility results were biased by being part of a rehabilitation programme at 3 months post-operatively.

Source	Design and participants	Intervention	Outcome measures	Results	Quality and comment
Heine et al (2004)	Qualitative study – grounded theory to explore service user perceptions Aim: participants' views of what factors contribute to a feeling of readiness for discharge if sent home 5–7 days post-operatively Purposive sampling of five participants from a single acute setting Age range 43–79 years Male:female ratio = 3:2 Australia.	Total hip replacement.	In-depth unstructured interviews – 30–75 minutes Due to be discharged in 1–2 days Prior to discharge participants were asked: 'When are you going home?' and 'Tell me how you feel about going home'.	Three major categories emerged from the data: a) Feeling safe b) Confidence c) Family and friends. These categories represented the general pattern of readiness for discharge, despite the discharge process being unique for each service user Service users need to feel safe or secure about their return home – can be enhanced by providing information at a pre-operative stage as well as prior to discharge.	Grade D – Very Low Limitations: • Essentially case study accounts • No pilot study and analysis reported all relevant topic areas covered after only five participants • No tape recording of interviews – field notes only • Not clear if researcher involved in treatment.
Hobbs et al (2011)	Cross-sectional cohort study Aim: to understand service user expectations of total hip replacement Recruitment via 20 orthopaedic centres across Europe Inclusion: diagnosis of osteoarthritis of the hip, primary total hip replacement (THR) and willing to participate 1,327 sampled (1,108 responses) 12 European countries.	Total hip replacement.	Used International Classification of Functioning, Disability and Health (ICF) as way of classifying service user expectations following open questions about their wants and needs after THR surgery Wants and needs were grouped into 3 categories of the ICF.	• Service user needs are different from their wants • Need expectations were classified as activity limitation • Want expectations were classified as activity limitation and participation restriction combined • THR targets impairment, but most patients expected and wanted improvements in disability-related outcomes, which could result in poor patient satisfaction results.	Grade C – Low Comments: • Lack of insight into confounding factors and exclusion criteria.

Source	Design and participants	Intervention	Outcome measures	Results	Quality and comment
Hol et al (2010)	Systematic review Aim: to determine whether immediate post-operative unrestricted weight-bearing may have an influence on bony consolidation and eventual loosening of uncemented femoral stem in total hip replacement Criteria: 1. THR for osteoarthritis 2. Intervention post-operatively full weight-bearing with aid 3. Primary outcome was osseous integration, loosening of subsidence and femoral migration. 13 studies: 10 RCTs, 3 controlled clinical trials.	Uncemented primary total hip replacement Full weight-bearing immediately post-operatively.	Degree of subsidence and osseous integration of femoral stem after THR and full weight-bearing protocol.	Subsidence of femoral stem – all occurred within the first 3 months and after that was stable Main result is that immediate unrestricted weight-bearing is not contra-indicated in people with primary uncemented THR Moderate – strong evidence for full weight-bearing immediately post-operative with uncemented THR – can allow quicker rehabilitation and return to functional independence Despite variety of methods study shows minimal risk of stem migration with full weight-bearing Supportive of accelerated rehabilitation programmes.	Grade B – Moderate Downgraded from Grade A due to limitations: • Not all studies were randomised controlled trials • Small sample sizes (range 23–80) • Pooling not considered to be feasible due to differences in studies • Use of assistive device and exact description of weight-bearing status unclear • Different methods of quantifying migration of femoral stem used.
Hunt et al (2009)	Qualitative study Aim: to describe service user experience of accelerated discharge after hip replacement in order to test the acceptability to service users of economically driven shortening of post-operative stay Belfast n=20 Mean age 70 years Male:female ratio 9:11 Liverpool n=15 Mean age 71 years Male:female ratio = 8:7 United Kingdom.	Total hip replacement Two groups from two hospitals: 1. Belfast – accelerated discharge programme, aiming for a post-operative stay of 3–4 days (cases) 2. Liverpool – traditional regimen of discharge after 6–7 days (controls).	Semi-structured interviews of service users' feelings and experiences relating to their intervention.	Service users primarily concerned with how attentive and informative hospital staff had been, and did not spontaneously refer to length of stay When prompted, they did not question their discharge time, though those with traditional care could not countenance more rapid discharge Service users with accelerated discharge described concerns about consequences of early discharge for them or their family – especially regarding managing pain and mobility problems at home and needing more support.	Grade D – Very Low Downgraded from Grade C due to limitations: • Differences in surgical, anaesthetic/pre-operative occupational therapy • Time post-surgery and interview length varied • Unclear if any researcher and participant bias • Small sample size • Awareness service users rarely criticise their care when asked overtly • Continuing inflammatory response at least 7 days after surgery: Liverpool sample (longer stay) response would be lower re feeling unwell at discharge.

Source	Design and participants	Intervention	Outcome measures	Results	Quality and comment
Husted et al (2008)	Prospective cohort study Aim: to identify service user characteristics associated with length of stay and service user satisfaction after total hip and knee replacement surgery Facility: dedicated fast-track joint replacement unit 712 unselected consecutive service users Mean age 69 years Male:female ratio = 272:440 Denmark.	Total hip replacement or total knee replacement with fast-track therapy and early discharge home within 5 days Standardised protocol throughout multidisciplinary team approach.	• Length of stay • Service user satisfaction (11 parameters via written questionnaire completed on discharge). 22 service user characteristics were examined.	92% discharged home in 5 days, 41% in 3 days. 88/712 didn't attend pre-operative meeting. No difference in LOS found between those who did and didn't attend, or between service users with different surgeons or operations at different times of day Age (older p=0.01), gender (females p=0.01), marital status (living alone p=0.02) had increased chance of staying longer than 3–5 days. There were similar outcomes for use of walking aids (p=0.004) and day of surgery (p=0.001) Study concluded that the accelerated discharge reduced LOS for unselected THR and TKR service users. High service user satisfaction was found for all parts of the stay with a readmission rate similar to other studies.	Grade C – Low Limitations: • Service user satisfaction tool not validity/reliability tested • No discussion on population specifics and what happens with complex service user discharge • No follow-up • No mention of outcomes for 8% who stayed more than 5 days • Difficult to determine generalisability of results.

Source	Design and participants	Intervention	Outcome measures	Results	Quality and comment
Ibrahim et al (2013)	Systematic review Aim: to present an evidence-based summary of some common interventions and methods in enhanced recovery in total hip replacement Inclusion: studies published in 10 years up to 2013 concerning Enhanced Recovery Programme and THR Exclusion: papers not published in English.	Non-surgical interventions: • Pre-operative education • Peri-operative haemoglobin (Hb) levels • Pre-operative patient nutrition • Pre-emptive analgesia • Local infiltration analgesia • American Society of Anaesthesiologists (ASA) grade • Pulsed electromagnetic fields (PEMF) • Peri-operative rehabilitation programmes • Post-operative hip precautionary measures • Dressings. Surgical interventions: • Conventional surgery and minimally invasive surgery • Fast-track joint replacement units.	Various outcomes measured, included: • Anxiety • Pain • Length of stay (LOS) • Recovery time.	Pre-operative education: • Makes service users active participants in their recovery and manages expectation • Individual pre-operative teaching can reduce LOS by one day • Reduces LOS and post-operative medication and anxiety • Pre-operative reduction in anxiety and pain • One study investigated pre- and post-operative education combined with home visits (compared with control receiving conventional rehabilitation) and found 4-day reduction in LOS and better Oxford Hip Scores. Peri-operative rehabilitation programmes: • Multidisciplinary teams that are highly organised tend to produce enhanced recovery and reduced LOS • Call to focus on early and more intensive physiotherapy after THR although varying evidence and outcomes with specific groups. Post-operative hip precautionary measures: • One study found a correlation between reduced LOS and a higher rate of dislocation after adopting pathways to reduce LOS.	Grade B – Moderate Downgraded due to: • Covered a large range of interventions, therefore depth of each study not explored • No discussion regarding quality of evidence included in review • Authors will receive benefits for personal or professional use from a commercial party related directly or indirectly to the subject of this article.

Source	Design and participants	Intervention	Outcome measures	Results	Quality and comment
Iyengar et al (2007)	Prospective cohort study Aim: role of targeted early rehabilitation at home for service users admitted for elective total hip replacement or total knee replacement – in terms of reduced length of stay (LOS), reduced cost, readmission rates, complication rates and costs of running scheme considered (cost-effectiveness) THR n=220 and TKR n=174 were eligible for rehabilitation at home out of total of 1,034 THR group: Mean age 72.1 years Male:female ratio = 42.7%:57.3% United Kingdom.	Total hip or knee replacement, early discharge with home-based multidisciplinary team rehabilitation Went home with service user on day of discharge and then saw service user in the home according to individual needs Screening in pre-operative clinic by occupational therapist to identify service users who could be discharged earlier with home rehabilitation if resources available in the community.	• Length of stay (days) • Duration of home rehabilitation (days) • Number of hospital bed days saved • Complications detected • Readmissions • Cost of home therapy programme.	• Targeted early rehabilitation resulted in reduced hospital stay (from 14 to 8.17 days for THR), without any increase in complication rates • THR service users had mean length of stay on rehabilitation scheme of 2.84 days. Targeted early rehabilitation at home after elective THA and TKA releases acute care beds and reduces healthcare costs No evidence of increased complication or readmission rates A multidisciplinary team working closely together was believed to be the key to success of the scheme.	Grade C – Low Limitations: • Need more information about the population of the study • Critical functioning criterion screening tool was not tested for validity and reliability • Targeted selection of service users – hence bias to shorter LOS • Long baseline LOS at beginning of study • Study did not compare with a similar selected cohort from the past.

Source	Design and participants	Intervention	Outcome measures	Results	Quality and comment
Johansson et al (2007)	Randomised controlled trial Aim: to determine whether it is possible to increase service user knowledge and certainty about care-related issues, to reach a more empowering learning experience and to exercise a more positive impact on selected clinical outcomes by additional pre-admission education 165 eligible, 123 participated Group A: n=62 Group B: n=61 Mean age 62.4 years Male:female ratio = 49%:51% Finland.	Total hip replacement Randomised to: • Group A – face-to-face education with nurses using the concept map method with written educational material • Group B – written education and non-systematic oral education (standard).	Data collected 4 weeks before admission, on admission and discharge: • Orthopaedics Patient Knowledge Questionnaire (OPKQ) prior to admission, on admission and shortened version on discharge • Modified Empowerment Questionnaire (MEQ) on admission • Clinical outcomes (length of stay, length of admission discussion and need for further care) – from medical record.	At 2nd post-test n=55(A); n=51(B) At first post-admission test Group A had significantly better knowledge and certainty of care-related issues (p=0.021) than Group B, as well as reporting more positive learning experience (p<0.001) In 2nd post-test at discharge – Group A had better knowledge and certainty of care-related issues (p=0.022) Pre-admission education using concept map method and written education yield better learning results than the use of written education material with non-systematic oral education. Written is more effective than verbal, should employ both strategies for pre-assessment.	Grade B – Moderate Downgraded from Grade A due to limitations: • Potential bias as Group B able to contact nurses as well • Both groups received education and even those who received only standard input had a good outcome • Proportion of drop-outs quite high at 27.
Johansson et al (2010)	Cohort study Aim: to examine impact of pre-operative functional status on early post-operative outcomes after total hip replacement n=75 Mean age: 67 years Male:female ratio = 39:36 Body mass index of <35 who underwent an uncemented THA for osteoarthritis Three surgeons involved, similar procedures Follow-up for at least 2 years Germany.	Total hip replacement Classified into three groups based on pre-operative Harris Hip Score – poor, intermediate and good.	Self-administered measures pre-operatively and at 6, 12 and 24 months: • Harris Hip Score (HHS) • SF-36® • WOMAC. Included pain, function, range of movement, quality of life, stiffness.	• Poor pre-operative Harris Hip Score is an indicator for poor early post-operative outcomes • Longer waiting times are detrimental to achieving the full benefit of surgery • Only pain and function (Harris Hip Scores) were significantly improved after THR at all time points for the evaluation (p<0.001) • Highlights importance of awareness of service users pre-operative Harris Hip Score in order to plan interventions and goal setting • Possible use of SF-36® and WOMAC measures.	Grade C – Low Limitations: • Exclusion criteria only account for select co-morbidities with no reason given for this. The presence of other co-morbidities has a possible confounding effect on results • Limited information regarding recruitment of cohort • No information how approached to complete the measures or about completeness of study (i.e. drop-outs over 24-month period).

Source	Design and participants	Intervention	Outcome measures	Results	Quality and comment
Judge et al (2011)	Prospective cohort study Aim: to identify patient characteristics associated with pre-operative expectations of total hip replacement, and whether those expectations predict surgical outcomes (pain, stiffness and physical function) 12 months post-operatively n=1327 THR in 20 European orthopaedics centres Mean age 65.7 years Male:female ratio = 44.1%:55.9% Europe.	Total hip replacement.	• WOMAC Score • EQ-5D™ Score • Outcome measures in rheumatology • Body mass index • Medication use.	Used Patient Reported Outcome Measures (PROMs) to evaluate success from the service user's perspective There is wide variation in service user expectations Service users with more pre-operative expectations are more likely to have clinically important outcomes 12 months post-THR (95% confidence interval) Service users who are younger, female, have a higher body mass index and higher level of education tended to have higher levels of expectation Greater numbers of pre-operative expectations are associated with improvement following THR.	Grade C – Low Limitations: • Unable to measure the importance attributed to different expectations by individuals • Does not consider the role of changes to lifestyle/behaviours in achieving expectations • Potential halo effect from the expectation question at the end.
Khan et al (2008)	Cochrane Systematic Review Aim: to assess evidence for effectiveness of organised multidisciplinary rehabilitation on activity and participation in adults (18+) following hip or knee replacement surgery for chronic arthropathy Included RCTs covering multidisciplinary rehabilitation with routine services, hip or knee joint replacement Five trials (n=619) met inclusion criteria – two inpatient rehabilitation (n=261) and three home-based settings (n=358) Studies: United Kingdom, Iceland, Australia and United States.	Total hip or knee replacement followed by multidisciplinary rehabilitation defined as: • Two or more disciplines involved • Home, hospital or outpatient • Early or late timing • Use of critical pathways • Use of pain management strategies. Control intervention – lower-level or different type of intervention, equivalent in a different setting or waiting list conditions.	• Impairment (e.g. joint range of movement and muscle weakness) • Activity limitation (e.g. mobility transfer skills, independence in activities of daily living) • Restriction in participation (e.g. extended activities of daily living, societal reintegration, quality of life). Others: cost of episode of care, length of stay, service utilisation, readmission, mortality rates, carer burden.	• No studies providing direct evidence that multidisciplinary rehabilitation following THR/TKR achieved better outcomes compared with no treatment • Evidence for the effectiveness of multidisciplinary rehabilitation in both inpatient and home-based settings • Not possible to suggest best 'dose' of therapy • Modest support that following hip replacement people should be assessed for need for appropriate rehabilitative intervention. Evidence that multidisciplinary rehabilitation programmes can have a positive impact on service user-related outcomes, such as function and quality or life, as well as institutional outcomes, e.g. length of stay and cost.	Grade A – High Limitations: • Studies themselves were low quality • Small numbers and methodological weaknesses • Difficulties with combining information due to heterogeneity of studies – could not perform meta-analysis • Best evidence synthesis using a qualitative analysis completed.

Source	Design and participants	Intervention	Outcome measures	Results	Quality and comment
Kiefer and Emery (2004)	Cohort retrospective review Aim: to measure functional gains in self-care, mobility and locomotion of service users after total hip replacement from baseline to discharge. Also compare grip strength to normative data in over 60 age group, and examine the relationship between grip strength and functional performance measures after THR Rehabilitation unit n=41 Mean age 72.9 years Male:female ratio = 13:28 United Kingdom.	Total hip replacement.	Functional Independence Measure (FIM™) Jamar Dynamometer Measures at baseline and discharge.	• FIM™ subscale scores improved 2.1 points on average. Statistically significant improvement made in 10 subscales of self-care, mobility and locomotion ($p \leq 0.05$) • Grip strength significantly less than expected norms in 6 of 14 sub-groups after surgery • No significant correlation between grip strength and FIM™ subscale (at 0.05). Improvement of functional performance made on all FIM™ subscales. Grip strength after THR was moderately decreased from the norm • Significant improvement in all FIM™ areas other than eating and cognition where score was independent at baseline ($p \leq 0.05$).	Grade C – Low Limitations: • Small sample size • Exclusion criterion makes it difficult to generalise – no upper limb issues • No pre-surgery measures to compare against • No control group to compare.
Kim et al (2003)	Literature review Critical review of evidence on clinical pathway effectiveness for total hip and knee replacement Study designs prospective, retrospective or randomised control trials with either historical or concurrent controls 11 included in review 10 historical, one concurrent RCT.	Use versus the non-use of clinical pathways following total hip or knee replacement.	Four outcomes: • Length of stay in acute facility • Total cost of acute hospitalisation • Complications (factors affecting recovery requiring readmission or variation from the clinical pathway) • Functional outcomes and pain (physician-administered, or service user-reported questionnaire).	Reviewers found that implementation of clinical pathways for total hip and knee replacement service users was associated with: • Reduced length of stay (LOS) and hospital costs • Reduced or unchanged rates of complications • Either improvement or no change in service user-reported outcomes. Evidence supported use of clinical pathways.	Grade B – Moderate Downgraded from Grade A due to limitations: • Pre-assessment/pre-operative input not considered • There is no evidence of a clear, pre-determined strategy or scoring system for full assessment of the quality of the studies • Failure to account for LOS in rehabilitation facilities • The use of historical controls in the studies creates the potential for bias due to secular trends in cost and resource use.

Source	Design and participants	Intervention	Outcome measures	Results	Quality and comment
Lin and Kaplan (2004)	Retrospective cohort study Aim: to explore which characteristics and factors are associated with increased length of stay at an acute rehabilitation hospital Single rehabilitation hospital n=808 Hip replacement (48%) or knee replacement Mean age 69.4 years Male:female ratio = 29%:71% United States of America.	Total hip or total knee replacement Rehabilitation in acute rehabilitation facility post-operatively.	Length of stay in acute rehabilitation facility (admission to discharge) Collection of data from database including a range of demographic factors, surgical factors and significant co-morbidities.	• Correlation between age and length of stay (LOS) – particularly for oldest group (p=0.004) • Gender (male p=0.055), co-morbid medical disease (p<0.001) found to be predictive of increased LOS • Marital status (single p=0.001) and race (black p=0.029) had influence in longer LOS • Body mass index makes no significant difference to LOS. The multivariate linear regression model used as a predictor showed that some relationships were statistically significant, but a poor predictor of exact length of stay in rehabilitation for an individual service user. It is more useful in examining groups of service users as a general guide to which groups may have increased LOS.	Grade C – Low Limitations: • Confounding variables (service user motivation in therapy; discharge destination and set-up; social needs and issues) • Data not available for transfer to other settings, rehabilitation facility, nursing care, etc. • The study acknowledges that they could only include factors that lent themselves to modelling – so aspects such as service user motivation and family issues were not included.
Malik et al (2002)	Case description Describes 3 service users who, in the immediate post-operative period, dislocated their THRs All 3 service users, 2 female and 1 male (aged 77, 40 and 64), underwent Charnley THR via the Hardinge approach. All had no cerebral dysfunction, no radiological evidence of component malposition and leg length discrepancies of less than 1 centimetre United Kingdom.	Total hip replacement.	Dislocation.	Service users dislocated at 14, 19 and 23 days post-operatively, when turning to answer the telephone. It was assumed that the dislocation was due to postural reasons The authors recommend that when discussing hip precautions and performance of activities of daily living post-operatively, specific mention should be made regarding the need to place the telephone in an easily accessible location, and think of safe limb positioning prior to automatically using the telephone without prior thought.	Grade D – Very Low Limitations: • Descriptive only • Case series but very limited information provided.

Source	Design and participants	Intervention	Outcome measures	Results	Quality and comment
Malviya et al (2014)	Systematic review Aim: to review literature on employed service users' expectations, highest risk for not returning to work, external factors that enable return to work, whether age determines ability/motivation to return, and ability to return at the same level Inclusion: qualitative and quantitative studies Exclusion: operations other than hip or knee replacement; living with osteoarthritis without consideration of total joint replacement; experience in primary care only or questionnaire development.	Total joint replacement – hip or knee.	Qualitative and quantitative literature was reviewed to determine evidence for the following questions: • What are the employed person's expectations from a joint replacement before and after surgery? • Who is most at risk of not returning to work after joint replacement surgery? • What external factors are important to help patients return to work? • Does age of the service user determine their ability/ motivation to return to work? • Are service users able to return to work at the same level?	• Barriers to employment are important factors driving patients to proceed with joint replacement surgery. Service users have high expectations of the impact of joint replacement on their ability to work, and unrealistic expectations lead to heightened frustration and slower rate of recovery • Service users who are unemployed before surgery are less likely to obtain gainful employment after surgery, and patients who have been off sick longer pre-operatively are less likely to return to work. Motivation is the key factor in early return to work • Good health and social care helps people return to work. • Service users on benefits are less likely to return to work, while those who are self-employed return to work sooner. Individuals who have no restriction on activity following joint replacement surgery return to work sooner • Younger service users and those with less co-morbidities are more likely to return to work • The majority of service users are able to return to work at the same level, although those involved in heavy manual labour return to work later, whilst those with light workload returned sooner.	Grade A – High Comments: • Search terms for qualitative studies very broad – this was due to the fact there were no results for qualitative studies examining work/ employment in people undergoing total joint replacement. A wider search was therefore conducted and data extracted from this • Average age greater than 62 years indicating working age individuals were not broadly represented • Selection bias suggested by the authors in the qualitative articles used.

Source	Design and participants	Intervention	Outcome measures	Results	Quality and comment
Mancuso et al (2003)	Cross-sectional design Aim: to measure service user pre-operative expectations of THR, and to assess whether expectations vary by demographic characteristics and functional status n=1103 Primary unilateral or bilateral THR Mean age 65 ± 13 years Male:female ratio = 43%:57% United States of America.	Total hip replacement – unilateral or bilateral.	Self-reported pre-operatively: • Hospital for special surgery total hip replacement expectations survey • American Academy of Orthopaedics Surgeons hip/knee module • SF-36® – general health scale.	Significant evidence that decreased status pre-operatively results in greater expectation of THR surgery and greater importance on post-operative achievement of goals Pain relief and improvement in walking were most prevalent expectations • Service users with worse hip function had more expectations compared with patients who had better hip function (p=0.0001) • Similarly, service users who had worse overall physical health had more expectations compared with service users who had better physical health (p=0.0001) • Service users with worse function were particularly more likely to expect relief of night pain and to not need medications compared with service users who had better function (p=0.001).	Grade C – Low Limitations • Allocation unclear • Possible bias through self-reporting • Co-morbidities not included in analysis • Single setting • Not controlled for severity of pre-operative condition • Unclear if differences existed in pre-operative discussion about expectations between surgeons and service users.

Source	Design and participants	Intervention	Outcome measures	Results	Quality and comment
Marks (2008)	Retrospective cross-sectional Aim: to examine if pre-surgical clinical presentation and short-term functional outcomes differ between service users' sub-groups undergoing hip joint replacement for end stage hip osteoarthritis Recruitment: records of 1,000 consecutive THRs. From this cohort 2 groups identified – non-traumatic and those with past hip fracture history n=42 in each group Male:female ratio = 17:25 No trauma group 72.28 years Trauma group 74.05 years United States of America.	Total hip replacement.	Pre-surgery: factors considered included body mass index, co-morbidity, duration of condition, pain, baseline hip flexion and internal rotation range of movement, pre-surgical walking status, leg strength Post-surgery: walking distance at 1 and 3 days.	Those with traumatic fracture history reported: • More frequent use of mobility devices and dependency on wheelchair • Pre-surgical device use more prevalent (p=0.023) and poorer ambulatory function and stair climbing ability (p=0.001) • Lower rate of functional recovery post-operatively. Overall suggests those with prior hip fracture history have longer duration of disability and are more functionally impaired pre-surgery (p<0.05).	Grade C – Low Limitations: • No evidence of any calculations to determine sample size • One hospital location and cohort over restricted time period • Retrospective self-reported data obtained from case records • Only one researcher extracted data • Short-term hospital-based outcome only • Some contradiction in results.

Source	Design and participants	Intervention	Outcome measures	Results	Quality and comment
McDonald et al (2014)	Systematic review Aim: to determine whether education pre-surgery for total hip or knee replacement improves post-operative outcomes Inclusion: RCTs or quasi-randomised trials of pre-operative verbal, written or audiovisual information delivered by a health professional within six weeks of surgery to people undergoing hip or knee replacement (elective) compared with usual care Exclusion: information not specific to surgery, comparing method of information instead of usual care, included post-operative intervention, investigating effect of pre-operative depression or recovery and didn't investigate post-operative outcomes 18 trials (1,463 participants) Mean age: 58–73 years Male:female ratio 41%:59% Hospitals in North America or Europe.	The format of pre-operative education ranged from one-to-one verbal communication, patient group sessions, or video or booklet with no verbal communication Delivered within 6 weeks of surgery.	Major outcomes: • Pain (visual analogue scales, numerical or categorical rating scales) • Function (WOMAC, Harris Hip Score, Oxford Hip/Knee Score, SF-36 Physical Component Score, Health Assessment Questionnaire, any other function scale) • Health-related quality of life (SF-36 or Nottingham Health Profile) • Global assessment post-operative anxiety (State-Trait Anxiety Inventory or Hospital Anxiety and Depression Scale) • Total adverse events • Re-operation rate. Minor outcomes: • Pre-operative anxiety (State-Trait Anxiety Inventory or Hospital Anxiety and Depression Scale) • Length of hospital stay • Mobility (number of days to stand or walk) • Range of motion.	For THR pre-operative education may not offer additional benefits over usual care: • Lower scores re anxiety, pain and function at various time frames post-operatively. Low quality evidence suggesting that pre-operative education may not improve pain, function, health-related quality of life and post-operative anxiety any more than usual care • Reduced pre-operative anxiety, but small effect and participants not blind to treatment • Reduction in length of stay non-significant • Reporting of adverse effects, such as infection, lower in pre-operative education group, but not significantly so.	Grade A – High Comments: • Low overall quality of evidence • Further research needed (especially regarding pre-operative education targeted at individual needs and optimal method(s) of delivery), which may have an impact on the confidence in the estimate of effect • Concern about risk of bias due to lack of blinding and imprecision of the effect estimates • Eight trials were rated as high risk of selective reporting bias because the data that was needed for a meta-analysis was not reported • Searches limited to electronic databases, therefore included only published trials • No mention of non-English language studies.

Source	Design and participants	Intervention	Outcome measures	Results	Quality and comment
McDonald et al (2004)	Cochrane review Aim: to determine whether pre-operative education improves post-operative outcomes (anxiety, pain, mobility, length of stay (LOS) and incidence of deep vein thrombosis) in service users undergoing hip or knee replacement surgery Randomised controlled trials or quasi-randomised trials 9 studies Total of 782 participants Variety of locations and services.	Pre-operative education delivered within 6 weeks of total hip or total knee replacement.	• Post-operative pain • Length of hospital stay • Compliance with post-operative exercise routine • Service user satisfaction • Deep vein thrombosis occurrence • Range of motion • Pre-operative anxiety • Post-operative anxiety • Post-operative mobility.	Insufficient evidence to support or refute the use of pre-operative education to improve post-operative outcomes, especially in terms of functioning and LOS • Insufficient evidence from available studies to support the use of pre-operative education over and above standard care to improve post-operative outcomes (pain, function and LOS) • May be beneficial effects when targeted at reducing anxiety, and for those most at need of support (greater disability and limited social support) • Moderate evidence that pre-operative education has moderate beneficial effect on pre-operative anxiety.	Grade A – High Limitations: • Small number of studies • Use of active comparator in most studies where control groups also received some form of pre-operative education also to result in smaller effect sizes than if control group had no input • Meta-analysis showed pre-operative education is beneficial in reducing pre-operative anxiety, but in the one case reviewed, effect was small and didn't support other research.

Source	Design and participants	Intervention	Outcome measures	Results	Quality and comment
McHugh and Luker (2012)	Qualitative research Aim: to understand service users' experiences post-total hip replacement (THR) Recruitment from a larger cohort participating in a longitudinal study Inclusion: osteoarthritis Main reason for operation was pain 25 participants Mean age 66.3 years Age range 48–82 years Male:female ratio=3:2 United Kingdom.	Total hip replacement.	Interviewed at 6 months post-operatively • Decision to have THR • Expectations of THR • Challenges of recovery • Supports for service users.	• Participants had high expectations for post-operative function that were not met • Pain was reduced • Patient Reported Outcome Measures (PROM) improved, but functional gains were not as hoped for (whatever age) • Fear of displacement/dislocation and falling was a challenge and often prevented patients from doing too much. Building confidence was an important theme • Lack of support from health professional re: how to progress their recovery • Limited physiotherapy post-operatively (up to 6 weeks) • Limited support for some participants • Limited rehabilitation options • Participants wanted more feedback and reassurance on how they were doing.	Grade C – Low Comments: • Small sample of 25 • Recall bias in remembering their experiences • Participants were part of a larger study that focused on functional outcomes – possible focus, therefore, on functional limitations • Lack of information regarding the relationship of researchers to participants and also lack of triangulation, explicit information about resolving disagreements about coding/themes between the two researchers could introduce bias and affect rigour • Also unclear about exactly how purposively sampling of participants from 215 available took place.

Source	Design and participants	Intervention	Outcome measures	Results	Quality and comment
McQuaid et al (2014)	Cohort study Aim: to evaluate outcomes of consultant-led decision to terminate routine use of hip precautions Recruitment via NHS foundation trust Inclusion: all service users who received total hip replacement, revision hip replacement or hemiarthroplasty between April and October 2013 100 participants Elective n=80 Average age: 60 years Trauma n=20 Average age: 78 years United Kingdom.	Consultant-led decision to terminate the routine use of hip precautions for total hip replacement 78 (97.5%) of elective and 19 (95%) of trauma did not use hip precautions.	How the use of hip precautions influenced an occupational therapy and orthopaedic service After 12 weeks a structured telephone interview was conducted by therapists Documented whether adaptive equipment was provided, how long this was used for, and whether hip dislocation occurred.	Dislocation: • Only 2 reported • Higher dislocation rate not associated with posterior approach. Equipment use: • Since removal of routine hip precautions, therapists' rationale for equipment mainly based on pre-operative pain management and functional ability • All participants received occupational therapy assessment and 89% required equipment for safe discharge. Precautions may impede recovery: • Therapists can discuss returning to activities without adaptive equipment • Imposing non-essential restrictions disables service users and creates dependence on equipment or carers. Length of stay: • Reduced length of stay for elective group from 7.1 days to 3.9 (though not solely attributed to removal of precautions) • Occupational therapists required to predict functional outcomes and equipment needs in order to have home environment prepared prior to surgery. This requires higher level of clinical reasoning and enhances the professional role.	Grade C – Low Comments: • Not all eligible to participate were willing or able to respond • Recall bias may have influenced the findings as patients were questioned 12 weeks after surgery • In some cases third party data was provided (if participants could not answer for themselves due to sensory or cognitive deficits) • Small sample and single service – cannot be directly replicated • In addition, the lack of separation of data regarding THR, revision and hemiarthroplasty is a limitation.

Source	Design and participants	Intervention	Outcome measures	Results	Quality and comment
Mobasheri et al (2006)	Cross-sectional design – retrospective Aim: to examine effect of THR on work status of service users under 60 years n=86 Service users post-operative between 6 months and 10 years Mean age 51.4 years Male:female ratio = 56:30 Questionnaire via telephone or in person United Kingdom.	Total hip replacement.	Questionnaire via telephone or at clinic post-operatively, items related to: • Profession • Employment status pre- and post-operatively • Length of time to resume work • Changes in working patterns • Reasons for not returning to work where relevant. Notes from pre-operative used.	Nearly all service users who were working pre-operatively returned to their jobs 49/51 Of the 30 who were not employed pre-operatively, 13 returned to the workforce 17 remained unemployed Only 12/30 who were not working pre-operatively were due to hip pain, therefore 18/30 had other reasons for not working. Of these 12, 11 returned to work post-operatively. Of the 19 not at work post-operatively – 5 were retired, 4 housewives and 10 reported they were not working for non-hip-related reasons Return to work rates were average 10.5 weeks for those working pre-operatively, and 35 weeks if not working pre-operatively.	Grade D – Very Low Downgraded from Grade C due to limitations: • Limited information on methodology • Length of time until follow-up (up to 10 years) possible bias in recall • Unclear if everyone responded • Single centre.

Source	Design and participants	Intervention	Outcome measures	Results	Quality and comment
Montin et al (2007)	Cohort study – longitudinal follow-up Aim: to identify whether service users undergoing THR for osteoarthritis were anxious and whether anxiety was associated with service users' health-related quality of life before and after surgery or with other background factors n=100 consecutively recruited Mean age 63.9 years Male:female ratio = 46%:54% Finland.	Total hip replacement.	Anxiety – measured by State-Trait Anxiety Inventory (STAI) Changes in health-related quality of life were evaluated by Sickness Impact Profile (SIP) Background, environmental and surgery factors.	Mean trait anxiety (STAI score) before surgery = 42.8 (Standard deviation 4.9). Age and pre-operative pain associated with trait anxiety, with a significant correlation ($p<0.001$ and $p=0.003$ respectively) Service users' anxiety increased slightly – not significant 3 and 6 months post-operatively Before surgery, older ($p=0.028$) and overweight service users ($p=0.030$) experience greater state anxiety A longer length of stay resulted in decreased anxiety post-operatively – significant at 3 months post-operatively ($p=0.020$) Pre-operative pain increases anxiety and reduces health-related quality of life after surgery – not significant statistically.	Grade C – Low Limitations: • No co-morbidities • One specialist hospital • Drop-out rate 13%.
Naylor et al (2008)	Prospective, cohort, longitudinal study Aim: to address two questions: 1. Are either severe other joint disease or obesity associated with a slower rate of recovery after total hip or knee replacement surgery? 2. Are they associated with less absolute recovery up to one year post-surgery? n=122 consecutive service users. At 52 weeks (55 knee, 44 hip) 99 remaining Mean age and male:female ratio depends on stratification Australia.	Total hip or knee replacement.	Measured 2, 6, 12, 26 and 52 weeks post-operatively: • Visual analogue scale for pain • 15m Walk Test • Timed Up and Go • Walking aid utilisation (at 52 weeks only) • Global improvement – using a five-level scale (taken at 52 weeks only). Subset questionnaires: • WOMAC • SF-36®.	Participants with severe other joint disease recovered more slowly in terms of mobility than the non-severe group ($p=0.005$). They also walked more slowly on the Walk Test, and took longer on the Timed Up and Go Test. They also had a greater chance of using a walking aid at 52 weeks (95% confidence interval) A similar profile was obtained for the obese compared to non-obese group Participants with severe other joint disease had significantly higher body mass index ($p=0.01$) and recovered more slowly (walking, stiffness, function). Rate of recovery in terms of pain and mobility were similar.	Grade C – Low Limitations: • Not possible to control for extrinsic influences: surgeon volume, etc. • Subset who completed additional self-reported outcomes not clearly identified • Lack of ability to blind the trial received but two observers trained to carry out the observation.

Source	Design and participants	Intervention	Outcome measures	Results	Quality and comment
Nickinson et al (2009)	Prospective cohort study Aim: to investigate the presence and rates of anxiety and depression in post-surgical service users Hip and knee replacement service users within a one-month period at specialist orthopaedics hospital n=56 Mean age 67 years Male:female ratio = 33:23 27 were undergoing THR (22 primary, 5 revision) United Kingdom.	Total hip or knee replacement.	• Anxiety • Length of stay. Hospital Anxiety and Depression Scale – score of ≥8 was deemed to be diagnostic Completed on the day prior to surgery, then on each post-operative day up to and including day of discharge.	Anxiety: • Post-operatively 17/39 anxious prior to discharge. No variables were significant predictors of anxiety ($p>0.05$) • Mean time point for development of anxiety 1.94 days. Service users most anxious at 2.47 days. Depression: • No subjects depressed pre-operatively – post-operatively 28 service users (50%) became depressed prior to discharge • Mean time point for development of depression 2.43 days • On day of discharge only three scores remained above diagnostic level for depression – suggests depression transient. Mean length of stay of 5 days for depressed or anxious service users (4 days for non-anxious/depressed patients).	Grade C – Low Limitations: • Small study sample limits applicability • Limited information re surgery • Responder bias • Service users not followed up after discharge • Not possible to separate out THR from TKR within final results and findings.

Source	Design and participants	Intervention	Outcome measures	Results	Quality and comment
Nunley et al (2011)	Retrospective, multi-centre study Aim: to determine if young, active service users return to work after hip replacement surgery. Also to investigate the impact of various modern implant types on return to work. Minimum 1 year post-surgery n=943 completed the survey (response rate 68.3%) 806 eligible for analysis Mean age 49.5 years Male:female ratio = 531:275 United States of America.	Primary total hip replacement Controlled for potential bias such as co-morbidities, post-operative complications.	Telephone interviews No formal standardised tools Telephone questionnaire comparing pre-operative and post-operative employment-specific and service user-derived outcomes.	• Most young active service users employed before surgery can expect to return to work (90.4%), most to pre-operative occupation • Mean time off work 6.9 weeks • 13 'permanently disabled' after surgery, none stated due to hip • Very few (2.3%) limited in their ability to return to work because of their operative hip • Dramatic decrease (significant difference) in the number of service users working with job restrictions prior to surgery compared with after surgery ($p<0.0001$) • 3.2% described some form of permanent job restriction post-operatively • 1.7% indicated unable to work at their usual job because of hip • Some statistically significant findings relating to age/gender.	Grade C – Low Limitations: • Potential for recall bias • Variations in centres, surgeons, implants and regional differences re jobs • Excluded cemented implants as less likely to be employed pre- or post-operatively • Respondents to surveys tend to be those more satisfied • More active service users selected.
Oberg et al (2005)	Mixed-study design – methods quantitative and qualitative Aim: to compare information obtained from three standard instruments, and with information acquired from an unstructured interview n=10 from the waiting list Age 50–80 years, no other disabling diseases Mean age 64.9 years Male:female ratio = 4:6 Sweden.	Total hip replacement.	Four outcome measures used: • SF-36® • FAS (Functional Assessment System of lower extremity dysfunction) • Canadian Occupational Performance Measure (COPM©) • Unstructured interviews.	• All instruments delivered important information on the functional and activity status of service users • All were responsive to change in function and activity after surgery • The interview strengthened validity of the instruments • All instruments showed a lower quality of life and reduced function and activity status before surgery, changes were statistically significant for most variables despite small numbers • After surgery service users showed increased quality of life, especially in domains related to bodily function, mobility and pain and individual areas of COPM©.	Grade D – Very Low Downgraded from Grade C due to limitations: • Unable to determine whether any exposure intervention bias • Confounding variables: differences in surgery, post-operative complications, rehabilitation regimes, etc. • Unable to determine whether any drop-outs • Small sample size • No other medical conditions.

Source	Design and participants	Intervention	Outcome measures	Results	Quality and comment
O'Donnell et al (2006)	Describes a formal consensus process, used to incorporate the scientific evidence and practitioner experience for the development of primary total hip replacement guidelines at a specific specialised orthopaedics tertiary care facility Rehabilitation team occupational therapists and physiotherapists took the role of leading and coordinating the process Canada.	Development of post-operative primary total hip replacement rehabilitation management guidelines Involved identifying gaps and inconsistencies, a literature review, development of a survey followed by a consensus meeting based on nominal group technique.	Survey addressed key areas, organised by prosthetic configuration and surgical approach These included: hip precautions, early functional activity (e.g. weight-bearing status in relation to activities of daily living) and later activity recommendations such as driving, gardening and various athletic endeavours.	The guidelines were developed in response to service user satisfaction data that identified a need for improved information relating to the resumption of usual activities They include positional precautions 0–6 weeks, and timelines for post-operative functional activities and the resumption of leisure activities.	Grade D – Very Low Limitations: Descriptive of consensus process to achieving hip precaution guidelines and therefore relevant to a specific locality.

Source	Design and participants	Intervention	Outcome measures	Results	Quality and comment
Ollivier et al (2014)	Cohort study Aim: to determine the level of sporting activity, predictive factors for participating in sports, and any correlation between sports participation and surgery satisfaction Recruitment via a single institution Inclusion: aged 18–75 years, osteoarthritis, avascular necrosis, developmental dysplasia of the hip Exclusion: revision surgery, post traumatic arthritis, contralateral total hip replacement (THR) or hip disease, knee surgery 571 individuals responded out of 815 asked Mean period post total hip replacement 9.8 years Total hip replacement: Mean age: 61.3 years Male:female ratio = 52%:48% France.	Total hip or total knee replacement.	Self-administered questionnaire to assess current participation in sport.	• 366 returned to sporting activity. Participants engaged in more low impact sports compared to high impact sports • Age, gender and BMI had no impact on post-operative exercise participation • Participants who reported higher Harris Hip Score pre-operatively were significantly more likely to participate in exercise post-operatively • 205 did not participate in exercise.	Grade C – Low Comments: • Recall bias/patient understanding of questionnaire • Only subjective measures.

Source	Design and participants	Intervention	Outcome measures	Results	Quality and comment
Orpen and Harris (2010)	Qualitative study: phenomenological approach Aim: focus on service user accounts of their perceptions and experience of pre-operative assessment prior to hip replacement n=10 (age 16 and over) hospital setting Age 53–85 years Male:female ratio = 4:6 United Kingdom.	Total hip replacement Home-based pre-operative occupationa therapy intervention Intervention areas: • Performance of ADL • Environmental considerations • Social considerations.	Semi-structured interviews No specific outcome measures used.	Five main themes generated: • Pre-operative equipment use increases independence, progress and confidence • Individual needs are better met through timely visits • Competent therapist home intervention offers reassurance regarding surgery • Knowing home environment is suitable increases confidence in planning hospital discharge after surgery • Levels of social support require pre-operative assessment.	Grade C – Low Well-conducted study Limitations: • Recall bias – difference in time periods between intervention and follow-up • Two service users suffered post-operative complications, which may have led to a more negative experience.
Ostendorf et al (2004)	Prospective cohort study Aim: to define minimum set of service user-reported outcome measures required to assess health status after a total hip replacement Focus on pain and activities of daily living function Recruitment via THR waiting lists, three hospitals n=147 (data for 114) Mean age 67.6 years Male:female ratio = 43:71 Netherlands.	Total hip replacement.	Self-reported measures pre-operatively, post-operatively at 3 and 12 months • Oxford Hip Score (OHS) disease-specific measure • WOMAC – disease-specific measure • SF-36® and SF-12® – general health status • EQ-5D™ – generic health-related quality of life measure.	All outcome scores showed significant improvement at one year ($p<0.001$) apart from SF-36® One year after operation very large effect sizes for OHS, WOMAC and physical domains of SF-36®/12 and EQ-5D™ Recommend use of OHS and SF-12® in assessment of THR At conclusion 114 included. Non-finishers were accounted for. Extensive results section on all the tools.	Grade C – Low Well-conducted study Limitations: • 33 participants lost for analysis data • Some missing data approximated • Floor and ceiling effect of tools • Possible bias with phone interview when needed.

Source	Design and participants	Intervention	Outcome measures	Results	Quality and comment
Pape et al (2013)	Case control study Aim: to detect any beneficial effects on length of stay of having interprofessional meetings Inclusion: undergoing total hip arthroplasty (THA), total knee arthroplasty (TKA) or uni-compartmental knee arthroplasty (UKA) between 1 October 2007 and March 2008 Control group: 75 THA n=38 TKA n=34 UKA n=3 Male:female ratio = 12:13 Mean age: 69 years Intervention group: 88 THA n=42 TKA n=36 UKA n=10 Mean age: 67 years Male:female ratio: 5:4 Denmark.	A daily interprofessional meeting: surgeons, nurses, occupational therapists and physiotherapists used a checklist in discussing barriers and focus areas for discharging service users following hip and knee replacement and made joint decisions about which healthcare profession should handle a given task.	Length of hospital stay.	A significant reduction in the length of stay in hospital in total hip replacement participants (from a mean of 4.1 days (SD 2.1) to 2.7 days (SD 1.4), $p< 0.05$) but not in knee replacement participants.	Grade C – Low Comments: • Sample size too small to offer statistical significance • Not an RCT (participant groups could not be separated) • Other factors may have contributed to reduction in length of stay (LOS) (there had been a continuous decrease in LOS in the hospital for THA/TKA and UKA over the past years).

Source	Design and participants	Intervention	Outcome measures	Results	Quality and comment
Parsons et al (2009)	Qualitative – descriptive phenomenological study Aim: to explore the lived experiences of service users with severe osteoarthritis of the hip or knee joint while awaiting joint replacement surgery Purposive sampling n=6 service users (three THR and three TKR) referred to National Health Service waiting list for primary hip or knee replacement Median age 68.5 years Male:female ratio = 3:3 Unstructured interviews United Kingdom.	Total hip or knee replacements.	Unstructured interviews.	Six themes: • Coping and living with pain • Not being able to walk (and difficulty continuing to work) • Coping with everyday activities • Body image • Advice and support available • The effect of their disease upon family, friends and helpers.	Grade C – Low Limitations: • Small sample (n=6) • Combines THR (n=3) and TKR (n=3).

Source	Design and participants	Intervention	Outcome measures	Results	Quality and comment
Peak et al (2005)	Randomised controlled trial Hypothesis: dislocation is more likely to occur in service users who are not placed on post-operative functional restrictions (PFR) following total hip replacement Randomised pre-operatively Of 630 eligible consecutive service users, 265 (303 hips) consented to be randomised into 'restricted' or 'unrestricted' group Restricted group n=152 Unrestricted group n=151 Mean age 58.3 years Male:female ratio = 139:126 United States of America.	THR – both groups: limit range of flexion, external and internal rotation, and avoid adduction during first 6 weeks Restricted group: to maintain abduction while in bed, used raising equipment, prevented from sleeping on side, from driving or being a car passenger Unrestricted group: not *required* to follow additional restrictions, could *choose* to use equipment for comfort.	Self-administered survey/diary to check compliance Completed surveys returned at first post-operative visit – 6 weeks after surgery Final survey at second follow-up visit about 6 months after surgery • Number of dislocations • Service user satisfaction related to maximised functional independence/resumption of roles • Length of hospital stay • Cost.	At 6-month follow-up, unrestricted group reported a much greater degree of satisfaction re return to pre-operative daily activities ($p<0.001$). 89.4% of unrestricted group believed recovery was easier than if restrictions applied Compliance with restrictions – high in both groups, but higher in restricted group. Basic restrictions for all service users in first 6 weeks believed by authors to be critical Anterolateral approach likely to be associated with a low dislocation rate. Removal of restrictions did not increase dislocation prevalence Length of hospital stay – no difference. 3.5 days average for each group Additional expenditure in the restricted group due to equipment costs.	Grade B – Moderate Downgraded from Grade A due to limitations: • Serious concerns re overlap of treatment received by intervention v control group • Did not examine 'no precautions' v 'precautions', as all service users were advised to limit range of movement for first 6 weeks, but intervention group had further restrictions • Low dislocation rate may have been due to surgical approach, etc. • Study only evaluated uncomplicated cases.

Source	Design and participants	Intervention	Outcome measures	Results	Quality and comment
Restrepo et al (2011)	Prospective cohort study Aim: evaluation of the incidence of early dislocation following primary total hip replacement, with the observance of a no-restrictions protocol Context of the development of practice guidelines n=2532 Mean age 63.2 years Male:female ratio = 1223:1541 United States of America.	Total hip replacement via direct anterior approach or modified Hardinge anterolateral approach No restrictions protocol post-operatively; i.e. service user able to move operated hip through range of movement if comfortable, no use of elevated seats, no abduction pillows, no restrictions from driving.	Number of dislocations in 6-month period post-operatively. Determined by physician diagnosis, and self-reported where service user unable to attend follow-up Analysis included age, gender, body mass index, co-morbidities, diagnosis at time of surgery and implant design.	Four dislocations occurred 0.15% (4 of 2,612 total hip arthroplasties) at a mean of 5 days post-operatively One dislocation was service user with history of dysplasia of the hip, two occurred while on the toilet (one with a previous hip fracture treated with a modular system) and one dislocation was idiopathic Conclusion that no restriction protocol did not result in an increase in early dislocation Suggestion that controlling for pre-operative planning, correct prosthesis selection, surgical technique and accurate component positioning may alleviate need for hip restrictions.	Grade B – Moderate Upgraded from Grade C due to: • Large sample size • Inclusion of individuals with co-morbidities • Only 6-month follow-up, but likely to capture most dislocations • Expands on earlier study by same authors. Limitations: • 146 lost at follow-up • Single institution • Senior surgeons operate • No information on other outcomes of surgery • Service users may have implemented own precautions • Can't generalise outside of anterolateral approach.

Source	Design and participants	Intervention	Outcome measures	Results	Quality and comment
Rivard et al (2003)	Case control study Aim: to determine difference in discharge destination and overall length of stay between service users having a total hip replacement receiving pre-operative assessment or teaching at home compared to pre-admission clinic n=268 (analysis 206) Intervention group: n=102 Mean age 66.97 years Male:female ratio = 39%:61% Control group: n=104 Mean age 67.4 years Male:female ratio = 41%:59% Canada.	Total hip replacement Group A – Intervention: pre-operative home visit 1–2 weeks prior to surgery – 1:1 teaching and assess home environment directly Group B – Control: attended pre-operative assessment clinic within 1–2 weeks of surgery. Received teaching in a group setting, and therapists relied on client/family reports for information about the home environment.	Discharge disposition Length of hospital stay.	No significant difference in either discharge disposition or length of stay between Group A and Group B Issues raised re the complexity of resource allocation and the importance of qualitative dimensions of care The study found that length of stay or whether the service users were discharged directly home was not affected by the location of pre-operative teaching As confounding variables controlled, could assume that any differences in outcomes post-operatively are as a result of the intervention differences.	Grade B – Moderate Upgraded from Grade C due to: • Well-conducted study with comparative groups of good size • Considered age, number of co-morbidities and living alone as variables that could impact length of hospital stay • Administered WOMAC – no significant differences between the two groups. Limitations: • Comparison depends on replication of teaching/ visits.

Source	Design and participants	Intervention	Outcome measures	Results	Quality and comment
Sankar et al (2013)	Prospective cohort study Aim: to evaluate characteristics of those returning to work following joint replacement Recruitment via 4 tertiary care centres between 2005 and 2008 Inclusion: 18–85 years old; working or on short-term disability pre-surgery; English proficiency sufficient for the self-report questionnaires; consented Exclusion: revision or hemiarthroplasty, TJR for trauma or malignancy, reported that they chose not to work, were retired, unemployed or on long-term disability 931 participants TKR n=170; THR n=190 THR male:female ratio=10:9 THR mean age: 56.1 years 63% of THR employed full-time pre-surgery, and 39% with highly physical work Canada.	Total hip and total knee replacement.	Questionnaire completed pre-surgery (including demographics and type of occupation) and at 1, 3, 6 and 12 months post-surgery Primary outcome – return to work (at 1, 3, 6 or 12 months post-surgery) Secondary outcome – Workplace Activity Limitation Scale (WALS) Pain and physical function were evaluated using WOMAC Likert-version 3.0 Higher demand activities were reported using the limitations subscale of the Late Life Disability Index (LLDI).	• 166 (87%) and 144 (85%) returned to work by 12 months following THR and TKR respectively • The average time to return to work following THR was 10.5 weeks • Early (1 month) return to work was associated with: male gender, university education, working in business, finance or administration, and low physical demand work • People with THR returned to work earlier • For both groups, less pain and everyday functional limitations were associated with fewer workplace activity limitations at the time of return to work.	Grade C – Low Comments: • Patient recruitment limited to those having surgery in tertiary-care academic centres • No specific times given of return to work (this was linked to time frames of data collection) • May be bias in estimates of models due to conditional confounding from entering demographic variables as a block, or exclusion of important variables • Sample size limitations limited the number of covariates that could be modelled in relation to return to work.

Source	Design and participants	Intervention	Outcome measures	Results	Quality and comment
Siggeirsdottir et al (2005)	Randomised controlled trial Aim: to compare the outcome in a group of service users who experienced a shorter hospital stay with pre-operative education (augmented with home rehabilitation and nursing) with that in a group of service users who were subjected to current practices in post-operative rehabilitation n=50 – random allocation to: Study group (SG) n=27 Control group (CG) n=23 Mean age 68 years Male:female ratio = 24:26 Iceland.	Total hip replacement Study group (SG): • Pre-operative education/training • Occupational therapy and physiotherapy follow-up at home • Daily outpatient nurse visits for as long as required • Provision of a telephone number to contact with any questions. Control group (CG): • Treatment according to the clinical procedures already in use.	Day before the operation and 2, 4 and 6 months after operation: • Function • Pain • Quality of life. This included: • Oxford Hip Score • Nottingham Health Profile (part 1) • Functional scores of Meurle d'Abuigne and Postel • Harris Hip Score • A general questionnaire was also used.	• Hospital stay for the study group significantly shorter than the control group ($p<0.001$) • All service users in the SG returned directly to their homes, whereas only 10/23 of the CG did • 5/27 in the SG and 11/23 in the CG developed a complication – not statistically significant • No statistically significant results of the OHS between the groups pre-operatively, but results were in favour of the SG post-operatively ($p=0.001$ at 6 months) • Health-related quality of life (NHP) increased for both groups after the operation. Overall score indicated a lower quality of life in the CG • No significant difference between groups on the HHS. Score was better for the SG both pre- and post-operatively.	Grade C – Low Downgraded from Grade A due to limitations: • Small sample size – insufficient power • No details re control 'conventional' treatment • Unequal distribution of numbers in groups at one hospital, deviated from original protocol • Different implants and surgical approaches at the two hospitals • The numbers of service users accounted for fluctuation • Lack of blinding • No separation of pre-operative and post-operative education together with home visits.

Source	Design and participants	Intervention	Outcome measures	Results	Quality and comment
Smith and Sackley (2016)	Cohort study Aim: to determine current practices in the provision of hip precautions and equipment following primary total hip replacement Recruitment via professional networks Inclusion: health professionals 170 health professionals: 87 physiotherapists 83 occupational therapists Represented 170 health trusts United Kingdom.	Total hip precautions and provision of equipment.	Online survey of 27 questions • Current practices of occupational therapists and physiotherapists on the provision of post-operative equipment and hip precaution advice following primary total hip replacement • Attitudes of occupational therapists and physiotherapists to these practices • Service user groups where these practices are modified or amended due to differences in circumstances or patient characteristics • Attitudes towards the conduct of research to assess the use of post-operative equipment and hip precaution advice following primary total hip replacement.	• 87% routinely provided equipment but only 54% felt should do so • Raised toilet seats, toilet frames and rails, and furniture raises were most commonly prescribed • 61% prescribed pre-operatively, mostly by occupational therapists • Advice on length of use of equipment varied (half reported 6 weeks while 40% reported 3 months) • Surgical protocol, therapy protocol and clinician's personal assessment top reasons for provision • 97% routinely advised on hip precautions, but 25% felt should not be routine. 79% said all service users advised on hip precautions with few exceptions, • 48% reported they would like to change current practice, mostly to make it more individual • Hip flexion, adduction and rotation most commonly advised against • The length of hip precautions most commonly varied from 6 weeks post-operatively (55%) up to 3 months (36%) • 75% reported occupational therapists provided information, with half doing this at a pre-operative education group.	Grade C – Low Comments: • Could have received information from two or more individuals from same service • Not all information provided in full table/graph format – some in discussion of results only • No mention of piloting the study • Self-selecting convenience sample • Did not approach specific orthopaedic services.

Source	Design and participants	Intervention	Outcome measures	Results	Quality and comment
Smith et al (2016)	Systematic review Aim: to assess effects of assistive devices, hip precautions education, environmental modifications and activities of daily living (ADL)/extended activities of daily living (EADLs) training for total hip arthroplasty (THA) service users Inclusion: RCTs, quasi-RCTs and cluster RCTs that evaluated the effectiveness of elements in 'Aim', >80% underwent THA for osteoarthritis, may have included other studies as long as THA results presented, all types of prostheses, fixation methods and surgical approaches Exclusion: Non-RCTs 3 trials 492 participants who had received 530 THAs Male:female ratio nearly 1:1.	• Hip precautions • Assistive devices • Activities of daily living training • Environmental modifications.	Main outcomes: • Pain • Function • Health-related quality of life (HRQOL) • Global assessment of treatment success • Reoperation rate • Hip dislocation • Adverse events. Minor outcomes: • Limitations in Personal ADLs for initial 6 weeks • Restrictions in EADLs and instrumental activities of daily living (IADLs) • Societal reintegration and discretionary activities • Length of stay • Cost-analysis.	Three studies included considered as low/very low quality evidence One study found no adverse effects to not providing hip precautions, equipment or functional restrictions One study had uncertain results with respect to hip precautions One study was uncertain whether post-operative education and rehabilitation service with early discharge improved function compared to conventional discharge and rehabilitation intervention in the community Overall unable to draw conclusions because of low quality evidence.	Grade A – High Comments: • Evidence is only generalisable following primary THA and those with anterolateral approach (so currently incomplete knowledge on whether the post-operative equipment and functional activity requirement is different dependent on surgical approach adopted) • No meta-analysis possible due to lack of studies with similar intervention comparisons • Limited number of included papers • Paucity of evidence on disruption to activities of daily living and levels of extended and instrumental ADL.

Source	Design and participants	Intervention	Outcome measures	Results	Quality and comment
Smith et al (2015)	Systematic review with meta-ethnographic analysis Aim: to review the evidence on attitudes, perceptions and expectations of physical activity post-total hip replacement (THR) and total knee replacement (TKR) Inclusion: investigated the attitudes, perceptions or expectations of people prior to or after THA or TKA towards physical activity. No service user group based on demographics, previous health, length of arthroplasty being in place or severity of pathology was excluded 13 articles reviewed 282 patients TKR n=144 THR n= 134 Mean age ranged from 59 to 76 years Male:female ratio = 4:7.	Total hip replacement or total knee replacement.	• Attitudes, perceptions and expectations of physical activity post THR and TKR • Facilitators and barriers for return to physical activity post-arthroplasty.	• Following joint replacement service users have low expectations to participate in more activity than prior to surgery • Limited evidence to suggest service users increase their activity levels post-surgery, but desired to regain the same level of physical activity levels pre-pathology • One study suggested individuals simply wanted to be out of pain and undertake normal daily activities • Facilitators included external engagement and support from peers and others who had THR, social integration, early recovery with pain relief and perception of physical activity as a 'personal enjoyment' • Most common barrier was lack of or conflicting information on recovery and expected capability, along with age and other co-morbidities.	Grade B – Moderate Downgraded due to: • Unclear layout and results, making it difficult to interpret • Review of qualitative data, not high-quality data such as RCTs. Comments: • Studies did not always differentiate between THA and TKA which affects the confidence with which results can be applied to guideline population.

Source	Design and participants	Intervention	Outcome measures	Results	Quality and comment
Soever et al (2010)	Qualitative study Aim: identification of the educational needs of adults having hip or knee replacement surgery Purposive sampling, self-selected service users at two hospitals – one academic, one community. Pre- or post-surgery. Hip replacement – two pre- and seven post-operatives n=15 Age range 23–89 years Male:female ratio = 2:13 Canada.	Total hip or knee replacement.	Semi-structured interviews Perceptions of educational needs related to joint replacement surgery Pre-operative or post-operative (3–6 months after surgery) No standardised measures.	Several themes relating to educational needs and factors affecting educational needs: Educational needs – topics of interest, e.g. knowing the team, condition information and management, access, pre-operative activities, preparing for admission, rehabilitation process, functional recovery and follow-up Factors affecting educational needs (why education is important) – fears, family information needs and expectations Suggests clinical checklist of educational topics for all stages.	Grade C – Low Limitations: • Large proportion of female compared to male participants • Joint replacement did not distinguish between hip and knee requirements.
Spalding (2004)	Qualitative study Aim: to gain understanding of how the pre-operative education process achieves beneficial health and wellbeing outcomes previously proven in research Recruitment: via NHS Trust Health professionals n=7 Service users attending pre-operative sessions run by the health professionals n=10 United Kingdom.	Pre-operative education session within 3 months of planned total hip replacement surgery Session for 2 hours Up to 12 service users per group Explanation, demonstration and opportunity for service user participation and questions.	Pre-operative education sessions observed 5 times Health professionals – interviewed twice via semi-structured interviews Team meetings – 3 observed Service users – 2 semi-structured interviews (30min each) 2 weeks after pre-operative class and 1 week post-operatively Service user evaluations Data coded for themes.	Themes identified focus on empowerment of service users. This was coded into the following areas: confidence, trust, control, responsibility, involvement, support, knowledge and understanding Empowerment enables service users to take responsibility for their post-operative needs through providing a relaxed educational atmosphere, encouraging responsibility and choice, providing information booklets and involving peers and carers for additional support.	Grade C – Low Limitations: • Limited peer examination due to time constraints • Service users given opportunity to make changes – nil made • Credibility through triangulation not achieved from programme documentation • Occupational therapy-specific contribution not identified • No information about age and gender of service users.

Source	Design and participants	Intervention	Outcome measures	Results	Quality and comment
Spalding (2003)	Qualitative study Aim: to gain understanding of how pre-operative education process is beneficial in reducing anxiety for service users awaiting total hip replacement surgery Recruitment: via NHS Trust Health professionals n=7 Service users attending pre-operative sessions run by the health professionals n=10 United Kingdom.	Pre-operative education session within 3 months of planned total hip replacement surgery Session for 2 hours Up to 12 service users per group Explanation, demonstration and opportunity for service user participation and questions.	Pre-operative education sessions observed five times Health professionals – interviewed twice via semi-structured interviews Team meetings – three observed Service users – two semi-structured interviews (30min each) 2 weeks after pre-operative class and 1 week post-operatively Service user evaluations Data coded for themes.	Service user education can make the unknown familiar and reduce anxiety through: • Being able to understand experiences that will be encountered during and after surgery – provide chronological experience of THR • Opportunity to meet staff who will be involved in care on ward – familiar face • Familiarity with environment.	Grade C – Low Limitations: • No details provided on the backgrounds of the health professionals and their involvement in the educational session delivery • No information about age and gender of service users • No standardised instruments used.
Stewart and McMillan (2011)	Critical literature review Aim: to investigate factors influencing dislocation for hip fracture service users who had undergone hemiarthroplasty or THR Only three studies found that focused on hip restrictions and dislocation rate – related to elective cases.	Total hip replacement and hip restrictions.	Dislocation rates.	• Talbot: hemiarthroplasty, anterolateral approach, hip precautions unnecessary • Peak: insufficient evidence re how necessary hip precautions are for avoiding dislocation, but consensus that surgical approach, surgeon skill, cognitive capacity and hospital volume have greater importance. Modifying precautions by reducing limitations seemed to benefit service users • Ververeli – for THR following fracture, dislocation rate higher than electives. No study available re the necessity of hip precautions to avoid dislocation with hip fracture. Cannot generalise from elective.	Grade C – Low Downgraded from Grade A due to limitations: • Not a full systematic review • Not all RCTs, plus flaws in studies • No summary of papers or methodology • Search strategy and appraisal details limited • Did not state how many assessors reviewed each study • Insufficient studies – all relate to elective cases each with their own weaknesses and approaches.

Source	Design and participants	Intervention	Outcome measures	Results	Quality and comment
Thomas et al (2010)	Case study/evaluation Aim: to determine the most frequent reasons for non-use of adaptive equipment prescribed by occupational therapists for service users returning home after THR Convenience sample: nine service users from three different hospitals Average age 66 years Male:female ratio = 6:3 United States of America.	Occupational therapy prescription of adaptive equipment following total hip replacement.	Semi-structured telephone interview carried out post-surgery varying from 3 months to 4 years after intervention Questions developed by researchers.	• 72% stated always used their adaptive equipment • 78% stated little or no inclusion in decision making about equipment. • 85% stated adequate instruction given on use • 51% felt improvement in their medical condition affected length of time using equipment • 57% expressed home environment influenced non-use of equipment.	Grade D – Very Low Limitations: • Audit/service evaluation • No standardised measures used • Small sample, limited information on recruitment • Period post-surgery varied extensively • Number of confounding variables not explored • American healthcare system – all equipment purchased.
van der Weegen et al (2016)	Systematic review and meta-analysis Aim: to assess the evidence on the effectiveness of lifestyle restrictions and precautions in prevention dislocation post-total hip arthroplasty (THA) Inclusion: discusses undergoing total hip replacement, RCTs and comparative case series, English, Dutch or German language 6 papers 3 RCTs, 3 cohort studies.	Use of hip precautions following total hip replacement.	Dislocation rate, patient satisfaction, quality of life, return to independence with ADL.	The dislocation rate in the restriction group was 1.5% compared to 1.0% in the unrestricted group Significantly better results for patient satisfaction, quality of life and function in the no precautions groups. Resumed activities significantly faster.	Grade B – Moderate Downgraded due to: • Only 6 studies with some confounding factors and high heterogeneity, so true effect may be different to estimate Comments: • Some studies changed multiple variables when comparing to previous practice or control group • No details about assessment/tool used to determine quality of studies • Not all studies provided same level of detail about precaution protocols.

Source	Design and participants	Intervention	Outcome measures	Results	Quality and comment
Ververeli et al (2009)	Randomised controlled trial Aim: to evaluate the safety and effectiveness of an early rehabilitation protocol for THR service users. Test possibility of accelerating service user return to activities of daily living by minimising post-operative hip precautions n=81, allocation to: Standard rehabilitation group n=43 Mean ages 57.4/59.8 years Male:female ratio = 27:16 Early rehabilitation group n=38 Mean ages 58.8/60.8 years Male:female ratio = 22:16 United States of America.	Total hip replacement surgery and allocation by random numbers tables to either: Standard rehabilitation group: Restriction on bending hip and crossing legs at thighs, used equipment, etc. for first month Early rehabilitation group: Instructed not to cross their legs at the thighs, but otherwise no restrictions. Could bend the hip when they were comfortable and ride in a car. No equipment.	Assessed at approximately 4 weeks pre-operatively, and at 1 month, 3 months and 1 year post-operatively Service users completed: • Short Form 12-question Health Questionnaire (SF-12®) • Harris Hip Score • Diary of the number of days until they walked with a cane, walked without a cane, drove and walked without a limp. Service users also instructed to write any comments regarding their level of satisfaction and status of recovery.	• Early rehabilitation group were faster to ambulate with only a cane (p=0.03, moderately strong effect 0.48) and walked without a limp sooner (p=0.003, strong effect size 0.70) • Overall correlation between number of days walked with and without any assistive equipment (r=6), and early rehabilitation group were also faster to walk without a cane (p<0.001, effect size strong 0.89) • Early rehabilitation group began driving earlier (p=0.02). Strong effect size of 0.72 • Harris Hip Score indicated both groups regaining full range of motions/functions at same rate • Results from SF-12® were found to recover with the same physical strength and mental stamina • No incidences of dislocation. Early rehabilitation protocol increased pace of recovery without increasing complications.	Grade B – Moderate Downgraded from Grade A due to limitations: • Small sample size/ underpowered to have full confidence in terms of detecting a margin of difference in hip dislocation prevalence • Single-centre study • Exclusions to service user enrolment • Service users who consented might be less at risk • Larger number of men • The mean age quite low • Concerns about the lack of blinding • Differences in physical therapy provision between the two groups.

Source	Design and participants	Intervention	Outcome measures	Results	Quality and comment
Vincent et al (2012)	Systematic review Aim: to examine the relationship between obesity/ BMI and physical function after total hip replacement Inclusion: studies reporting a functional measurement of mobility, ambulation or transfers or a comprehensive self-report tool that assesses physical function, minimum of 6 months of follow-up after surgery; giving estimates of obesity; including surveys reflecting perceived physical functional ability; studies including functional tests Exclusion: less than 6 months' follow-up, studies not reporting functional measure or obesity assessment 23 articles Sample sizes ranged from 108 to 18,968.	Total hip replacement.	Functional outcomes – including: • Oxford Hip Score (OHS) • Harris Hip Score (HHS) • Western Ontario and McMaster Osteoarthritis Index (WOMAC) score • University of California, Los Angeles (UCLA) hip scoring system).	• Surgical approach did not affect outcomes for obese patients • 16 studies found obesity was associated with lower hip function at follow-up, though 4 did not • 5 studies revealed negative long-term effects of obesity on function, and one study noted no adverse influence of obesity on walking ability • Though obese patients do not achieve the same long-term functional level as non-obese counterparts, they have significant pain relief and satisfaction • Evidence does not show that reduced pain following surgery led to weight loss through increased activity.	Grade B – Moderate Downgraded due to: • Several studies demonstrated variability in the follow-up time points for assessment, which limits generalisability of the findings • Variations in surgical technique, component type and use of cement, and only a few studies controlled the number of surgeons • The determination of 'physical function' varied widely – no standard test battery • The reviewed studies did not report severity or frequency of other musculoskeletal pain that might be affected by THA • A substantial attrition rate occurred in many studies (creating selection bias) and it was not clear how missing data was handled.

Source	Design and participants	Intervention	Outcome measures	Results	Quality and comment
Vincent et al (2007)	Retrospective comparative study Aim: does obesity affect inpatient rehabilitation outcomes after total hip replacement? 178 medical records analysed Subjects stratified into four groups: Non-obese n=46 Overweight n=62 Obese n=50 Severely obese n=19 Gender and age varied across the groups United States of America.	Total hip replacement Interdisciplinary rehabilitation programme – 3 hours of daily supervised therapy from physical and occupational therapists Occupational therapists instructed activities of daily living for 30–45 minutes in the morning Group session of upper extremity activity Additionally three times a week advanced activities of daily living.	Data analysed against: • Functional independence FIM™ scores (at admission and on discharge) • Length of stay • FIM™ efficiency scores (change in FIM™ score divided by length of stay) • Hospital charges • Discharge disposition location.	• Revision THR service users had lower FIM™ score on admission and discharge • Changes in FIM™ scores between admission and discharge were not significantly different between four sub-groups ($p>0.05$) • Length of stay was significantly greater in the severely obese group compared with the non-obese group ($p<0.05$) • FIM™ efficiency scores were found to be lower in severely obese ($p<0.05$) • Non-obese and severely obese service users were less frequently discharged to home (non-obese had some co-morbidities) • Body mass index influences the outcomes of THR service users during inpatient rehabilitation.	Grade C – Low Limitations: • No information about surgical approaches • Not clear which service users were new referrals and which were THR revisions • Study did not attempt to match all subjects and control for confounders • Some occupational therapy interventions not transferable to UK setting (ball bouncing, stretching).

Source	Design and participants	Intervention	Outcome measures	Results	Quality and comment
Vissers et al (2013)	Cohort study Aim: to assess whether patients move actively at 4 years post-operation Exclusion for original study: >80 years old, wheelchair dependent, not living independently, planned total hip replacement (THR) or total knee replacement (TKR) within 6 months on other side, co-morbidities other than osteoarthritis that could affect function, residing more than 1½ hours from medical centre, insufficient understanding of the Dutch language Exclusion for this study: had TKR or THR in the previous 12 months, revision of a primary TKR or THR, or co-morbidities affecting function 44 participants THR n=23 TKR n=42 Had been involved in a previous study, which had initially recruited 77 patients Mean age: 63.8 years Male:female ratio = 18:26 Holland.	Total hip replacement and total knee replacement.	• Actual daily activity level at 4 years post-THR/TKR • Automated physical function data recorder • Hip disability and osteoarthritis outcome score • Knee injury and osteoarthritis outcome score • Automated sit to stand and mobility data recorder.	Actual daily activity had not increased between 6 months and 4 years post-operatively Functional capacity and perceived physical function had increased in same time frame Perception of improvement is better than actual activities of daily living (ADL) performance, which had not changed.	Grade C – Low Comments: • Limited scope • Large subjective element • Low sample number • Loss of patients to 4-year follow-up • Data only recorded for 48 hours.

Source	Design and participants	Intervention	Outcome measures	Results	Quality and comment
Wagenmakers et al (2011)	Cohort study Aim: to understand the physical activity and fulfilment of guidelines for health-enhancing physical activity for THA service users one-year post surgery Recruitment via 3 centres Inclusion: admitted for primary total hip replacement (THR) due to osteoarthritis Exclusion/attrition: death, other lower limb arthroplasty in the follow-up period, cognitive impairment 653 participants Mean age: 70.3 years Male:female ratio = 1:3 Netherlands.	Total hip replacement.	1 year follow-up, self-report questionnaire on level and intensity of physical activity.	• Participants aged over 75 years had lower activity and activity intensity than those under 75 • Participants with higher BMI had lower activity levels • Dislocation rate was 1.2% • Younger, fitter participants with lower BMI met the guideline level of activity more than those who were older, had more co-morbidities and higher BMI.	Grade C – Low Comments: • Selection bias due to non-response • Only used self-report questionnaires • Not clear the extent of generalisability • Definition of 'activity' unclear • Activity categories pre-determined.
Wang and Emery (2002)	Literature review Focus on cognitive status and its effect on recovery of functional performance following hip replacement Examined evaluation instruments to measure cognition and occupational therapy intervention to promote functional performance and how it is influenced by cognitive status 'Older people' not defined United States of America.	Total hip replacement and interventions to promote functional performance Occupational therapy – training and practice with adaptive equipment, education related to hip precautions and activities of daily living directed intervention.	Functional performance – no details of standardised outcome measures looking at functional performance Four measures to evaluate cognition: • MMSE – Mini mental status examination • Functional Independence Measure – cognitive subscale • SPMSQ – Short Portable Mental State Questionnaire • ACL – Allen Cognitive Level.	Importance of assessment of cognitive function as it affects success in pre-operative education, self-care and functional transfers The ability to learn about precautions and use adaptive equipment may be affected by cognitive status.	Grade C – Low Limitations: • Review not considered systematic and design of studies included could not be determined – assumption has to be made that these were mixed methodologies • No details provided for the literature review strategy • No assessment of the quality of the studies.

Source	Design and participants	Intervention	Outcome measures	Results	Quality and comment
Wang et al (2010)	Prospective cohort study Aim: to investigate factors affecting the short-term outcome of primary total hip replacement and develop a multivariate regression equation to predict the short-term outcome Elective primary total hip replacement – single service 82% had concurrent pre-operative co-morbidities n=97 (101 THR) Mean age 61.65 years Male:female ratio = 35:65 United States of America.	Total hip replacement Four surgeons involved.	Self-administered WOMAC at enrolment, 3 months, 1 year and 2 years post-operatively.	Statistically significant measure that indicates three main factors in predicting THR outcomes: pre-operative WOMAC Physical Function Score (p=0.0001), gender (p=0.0159) and pre-operative co-morbidities (p=0.0246) Predictive model derived and trialled; however, needs further study on its validity to THR Service users with better pre-operative functional scores likely to have higher post-operative scores, and service users with poorer pre-operative scores likely to experience greater improvement in function.	Grade C – Low Limitations: • Sample size – only 101 hips in regression analysis • Have not stated what is meant by outcome post-operatively, e.g. independent, working, back to normal • The pre-operative WOMAC scores had a large standard deviation therefore possible decrease in accuracy of prediction.
Williams et al (2012)	Retrospective cohort study Aim: to identify pre-operative factors that influence post-operative sports participation for individuals following total hip or total knee replacement 736 participants THA n=487 Mean age: 63 years Male:female ratio = 13:11 TKA=249 Mean age: 67.5 years Male:female ratio = 9:15 United States of America.	• Hip replacement metal on metal, metal on plastic, hip resurfacing, hip revision • Total knee replacement, uni-compartmental knee replacement, knee revision.	• Primary outcome was rate of sports participation at 1 year post-operatively using UCLA activity score • Compared demographics and surgical considerations.	• BMI, male, younger age and pre-operative UCLA activity score were predictors for higher post-operative UCLA activity score • Operation, surgeon, pre-operative WOMAC, Oxford Hip Score, SF-12 did not predict post-operative sports participation.	Grade C – Low Comments: • 46% response rate from total population and only 56% of these returned questionnaire at year one. • More active/motivated individuals may have replied • Definition of sports participation not clearly specified.

Source	Design and participants	Intervention	Outcome measures	Results	Quality and comment
Wilson and Villar (2011)	Expert opinion with some literature review Aim: to report advances in hip replacement surgery to cater for sporting patients and whether they return to sport post-THR United Kingdom.	Total hip replacement.	Level of return to sport.	Authors suggest: • It is important to manage patient expectations pre-operatively • Return to sport is possible • High impact/loading onto the hip will compromise the joint replacement • Selecting the right implant based on service user's planned activities is key • More research needed to see developments in new technologies that can cope with demands of sporting individuals, and evidence these technologies are reliable in the long term.	Grade D – Very Low Comments: • Small review of literature • Limited definitions or detail of sporting activities • Largely opinion based – more evidence needed throughout the article.
Wong et al (2002)	Prospective study Aim: to describe the hospital recovery pattern of older confused and non-confused service users after hip surgery Recruitment: consecutive admissions to a teaching hospital for emergency/elective hip surgery n=54 (not confused on admission) 28 admitted for osteoarthritis, 4 for revision THR and 22 fractured neck of femur Mean age 75.6 years Male:female ratio = 19:35 Canada.	Hip surgery – both elective and trauma Measurement of the effect of post-operative acute confusion on recovery pattern of older confused and non-confused service users after hip surgery.	Assessed at baseline and on first 4 post-operative days • Cognitive status (using Confusion Assessment Method) • Physiological status • Functional ability (Katz index of Activities of Daily Living) • Sleep satisfaction (using adapted form of Bowan's method) • Perceived discomfort (Discomfort Scale-Dementia Alzheimer Type). Length of stay (LOS) examined in context of acute confusion.	Older confused and non-confused service users recover from hip surgery differently. Majority of service users who developed acute confusion were hospitalised for fractured neck of femur • Of 54 service users, at least 12 (23%) developed acute confusion at some point after surgery • Confused and non-confused differed significantly in age, admission diagnosis and LOS ($p<0.005$) • Non-confused service users significantly more independent in activities of daily living • Confused service users had longer LOS ($p=0.0039$) • Both groups showed consistent improvement in functional status over time, but improvement of non-confused group is of greater magnitude ($p<0.005$).	Grade C – Low Limitations: • Replication of this study with a larger sample size needed to confirm findings • Inadequate instruments and methods used to evaluate discomfort and sleep satisfaction • Limited information about outcome measures (reliability and validity) • Analysis does not permit THR to be separated from fractured neck of femur – lack of details re variations in surgery • Longer follow-up period may have resulted in more definitive results.

Appendix 8: Glossary and abbreviations

AIMS	**Arthritis Impact Measurement Scale** Self-administered scales covering physical, social and emotional wellbeing, providing an indicator of the outcome of care for people with arthritis.
BAOT	**British Association of Occupational Therapists** The professional body for all occupational therapy staff in the United Kingdom.
CASP	**Critical Appraisal Skills Programme** Programme aiming to support the development of skills in the critical appraisal of scientific research, which provides a number of critical appraisal tools to support this activity.
COPM©	**Canadian Occupational Performance Measure** An individualised outcome measure which is designed to detect change in an individual's self-perception of their occupational performance over time.
CSI	**Caregiver Strain Index** Robinson's index consisting of 13 items that describe stressful aspects of caring.
EQ-5D™	**Generic health status measure** A standardised instrument for use as a measure of health outcome, providing a descriptive profile and a single index value for health status.
EQ-VAS	**Visual Analogue Scale component of the EQ-5D™** Records an individual's self-rated health on a visual analogue scale.
FAS	**Functional Assessment System of lower extremity dysfunction** An instrument designed for physiotherapists to evaluate lower limb problems focusing on hip, knee, functional and social variables and pain.
FIM™	**Functional Independence Measure** An 18-item ordinal scale, which measures independent performance in self-care, sphincter control, transfers, locomotion, communication and social cognition.
HAD	**Hospital Anxiety and Depression Scale** A screening tool, which measures separately the severity of anxiety and depression.
HHS	**Harris Hip Score** A disease-specific measure covering four domains of pain, function, deformity and motion.
LOS	**Length of stay** Period of time from admission into hospital to discharge.

OHS	**Oxford Hip Score** A short 12-item self-administered outcome tool to assess function and pain for people undergoing total hip replacement.
PROMs	**Patient Reported Outcome Measures** Measures to provide information on an individual's perceptions of the effectiveness of care delivered in the National Health Service.
RCOT	**Royal College of Occupational Therapists** A wholly owned subsidiary of BAOT operating as a registered charity. The College sets the professional and educational standards for the occupational therapy profession and represents the profession at the national and international levels.
RCOTTSS – Trauma and Orthopaedics	**Royal College of Occupational Therapists Specialist Section – Trauma and Orthopaedics** A branch of RCOT that promotes best practice in occupational therapy within the specialty of trauma, orthopaedics and rehabilitation of amputees.
RCT	**Randomised controlled trial** An experimental study in which the participants are randomly allocated to two or more different intervention groups, usually either the treatment of interest (intervention) group or the control (usual treatment) group.
SF-36®	**Health survey** A 36-question health survey which produces an 8-scale profile of functional health and wellbeing scores as well as psychometrically based physical and mental health summary measures and a preference-based health utility index.
SF-12®	**Health survey** Shortened version of SF-36®.
THR/THA	**Total hip replacement/Total hip arthroplasty** A surgical procedure in which a damaged hip joint is replaced with an artificial one (known as prosthesis).
TKR/TKA	**Total knee replacement/Total knee arthroplasty** A surgical procedure in which a damaged, worn or diseased knee joint is replaced with an artificial one.
UCLA	**University of California, Los Angeles Activity Scale** A scale to self-report current activity level; 1 defined as no physical activity, dependent on others and 10 defined as regular participation in impact sports.
WOMAC	**Western Ontario and McMaster Universities Osteoarthritis Index** A self-administered disease-specific, health status measure covering pain, stiffness and physical function in people with hip or knee osteoarthritis.

References

Evidence references

Aasvang EK, Luna IE, Kehlet H (2015) Challenges in postdischarge function and recovery: the case of fast-track hip and knee arthroplasty. *British Journal of Anaesthesia, 115(6),* 861–866.

Abe H, Sakai T, Nishii T, Takao M, Nakamura N, Sugano N (2014) Jogging after total hip arthroplasty. *The American Journal of Sports Medicine, 42(1),* 131–137.

Alviar MJ, Olver J, Brand C, Hale T, Khan F (2011) Do patient-reported outcome measures used in assessing outcomes in rehabilitation after hip and knee arthroplasty capture issues relevant to patients? Results of a systematic review and ICF linking process. *Journal of Rehabilitation Medicine, 43(5),* 374–381.

Arshad H, Royan S, Smith T, Barker L, Chirodian N, Wimhurst J (2014) Norwich Enhanced Recovery Programme vs non-enhanced recovery following hip and knee replacement: a matched cohort. *International Journal of Orthopaedic and Trauma Nursing, 18(4),* 227–234.

Barnsley L, Barnsley L, Page R (2015) Are hip precautions necessary post total hip arthroplasty? A systematic review. *Geriatric Orthopaedic Surgery and Rehabilitation, 6(3),* 230–235.

Berend KR, Lombardi Jr AV, Mallory TH (2004) Rapid recovery protocol for peri-operative care of total hip and total knee arthroplasty patients. *Surgical Technology International, 13,* 239–247.

Berge DJ, Dolin SJ, Williams AC, Harman R (2004) Pre-operative and post-operative effect of a pain management programme prior to total hip replacement: a randomized controlled trial. *Pain, 110(1–2),* 33–39.

Bohm ER (2010) The effect of total hip arthroplasty on employment. *The Journal of Arthroplasty, 25(1),* 15–18.

Bottros J, Klika AK, Milidonis MK, Toetz A, Fehribach A, Barsoum WK (2010) A rapid recovery programme after total hip arthroplasty. *Current Orthopaedics Practice, 21(4),* 381–384.

Brunenberg DE, van Steyn MJ, Sluimer JC, Bekebrede LL, Bulstra SK, Joore MA (2005) Joint Recovery Programme versus usual care: an economic evaluation of a clinical pathway for joint replacement surgery. *Medical Care, 43(10),* 1018–1026.

Caracciolo B, Giaquinto S (2005) Self-perceived distress and self-perceived functional recovery after recent total hip and knee arthroplasty. *Archives of Gerontology and Geriatrics, 41(2),* 77–81.

Chow WH (2001) An investigation of carers' burden: before and after a total hip replacement. *British Journal of Occupational Therapy, 64(10),* 503–508.

Coole C, Edwards C, Brewin C, Drummond A (2013) What do clinicians think about hip precautions following total hip replacement? *British Journal of Occupational Therapy, 76(7),* 300–307.

Coudeyre E, Jardin C, Givron P, Ribinik P, Revel M, Rannou F (2007) Could preoperative rehabilitation modify post-operative outcomes after total hip and knee arthroplasty? Elaboration of French clinical practice guidelines. *Annales de Réadaptation et de Médecine Physique, 50(3),* 189–197.

Cowie JG, Turnball GS, Ker AM, Breusch SJ (2013) Return to work and sports after total hip replacement. *Archives of Orthopaedic and Trauma Surgery, 133(5),* 695–700.

Crowe J, Henderson, J (2003) Pre-arthroplasty rehabilitation is effective in reducing hospital stay. *Canadian Journal of Occupational Therapy, 70(2),* 88–96.

de Groot IB, Bussmann HJ, Stam HJ, Verhaar JA (2008) Small increase of actual physical activity 6 months after total hip or knee arthroplasty. *Clinical Orthopaedics and Related Research, 466(9),* 2201–2208.

Drummond A, Coole C, Brewin C, Sinclair E (2012) Hip precautions following primary total hip replacement: a national survey of current occupational therapy practice. *British Journal of Occupational Therapy, 75(4),* 164–170.

Drummond A, Edwards C, Coole C, Brewin C (2013) What do we tell patients about elective total hip replacement in the UK? An analysis of patient literature. [Online] *BMC Musculoskeletal Disorders, 14(152),* 1–6. Available at: *http://www.biomedcentral.com/1471-2474/14/152*

Fielden JM, Scott S, Horne JG (2003) An investigation of patient satisfaction following discharge after total hip replacement surgery. *Orthopaedic Nursing, 22(6),* 429–436.

Gillen G, Berger SM, Lotia S, Morreale J, Siber MI, Trudo WJ (2007) Improving community skills after lower extremity joint replacement. *Physical and Occupational Therapy in Geriatrics, 25(4),* 41–54.

Grant S, St John W, Patterson E (2009) Recovery from total hip replacement surgery: 'It's not just physical'. *Qualitative Health Research, 19(11),* 612–620.

Harding P, Holland A, Delany C, Hinman R (2014) Do activity levels increase after total hip and knee arthroplasty? *Clinical Orthopaedics and Related Research, 472(5),* 1502–1511.

Heiberg KE, Ekeland A, Mengshoel AM (2013) Functional improvements desired by patients before and in the first year after total hip arthroplasty. [Online] *BMC Musculoskeletal Disorders, 14(243),* 1–8. Available at: *http://www.biomedcentral.com/1471-2474/14/243*

Heine J, Koch S, Goldie P (2004) Patients' experiences of readiness for discharge following a total hip replacement. *Australian Journal of Physiotherapy, 50(4),* 227–233.

Hobbs N, Dixon D, Rasmussen S, Judge A, Dreinhöfer, Günther KP, Dieppe P (2011) Patient preoperative expectations of total hip replacement in European orthopedic centers. *Arthritis Care and Research, 63(11),* 1521–1527.

Hol AM, van Grinsven S, Lucas C, van Susante JL, van Loon CJ (2010) Partial versus unrestricted weight bearing after an uncemented femoral stem in total hip arthroplasty: recommendation of a concise rehabilitation protocol from a systematic review of the literature. *Archives of Orthopaedics and Trauma Surgery, 130(4),* 547–555.

Hunt GR, Hall GM, Murthy BVS, O'Brien S, Beverland D, Lynch MC, Salmon P (2009) Early discharge following hip arthroplasty: patients' acceptance masks doubts and concerns. *Health Expectations, 12(2),* 130–137.

Husted H, Holm G, Jacobsen S (2008) Predictors of length of stay and patient satisfaction after hip and knee replacement surgery: fast-track experience in 712 patients. *Acta Orthopaedicsa, 79(2),* 168–173.

Ibrahim MS, Twaij H, Giebaly DE, Nizam I, Haddad FS (2013) Enhanced recovery in total hip replacement. *The Bone and Joint Journal, 95-B(12),* 1587–1594.

Iyengar KP, Nadkarni JB, Ivanovic N, Mahale A (2007) Targeted early rehabilitation at home after total hip and knee joint replacement: does it work? *Disability & Rehabilitation, 29(6),* 495–502.

Johansson HR, Bergschmidt P, Skripitz R, Finze S, Bader R, Mittelmeier W (2010) Impact of preoperative function on early postoperative outcome after total hip arthroplasty. *Journal of Orthopaedic Surgery, 18(1),* 6–10.

Johansson K, Salantera S, Katajisto J (2007) Empowering orthopaedics patients through preadmission education: results from a clinical study. *Patient Education and Counselling, 66(1),* 84–91.

Judge A, Cooper C, Arden NK, Williams S, Hobbs N, Dixon D. . .Dieppe PA (2011) Pre-operative expectation predicts 12-month post-operative outcome among patients undergoing primary total hip replacement in European orthopaedics centres. *Osteoarthritis and Cartilage, 19(6),* 659–667.

Khan F, Ng L, Gonzalez S, Hale T, Turner-Stokes L (2008) *Multidisciplinary rehabilitation programmes following joint replacement at the hip and knee in chronic arthropathy.* (Cochrane Review). Chichester, UK: John Wiley & Sons, Ltd. Available at: *http://onlinelibrary.wiley.com/doi/10.1002/14651858.CD004957.pub3/pdf*

Kiefer DE, Emery LJ (2004) Functional performance and grip strength after total hip replacement. *Occupational Therapy in Health Care, 18(4),* 41–56.

Kim S, Losina E, Solomon DH, Wright J, Katz JN (2003) Effectiveness of clinical pathways for total knee and total hip arthroplasty: literature review. *The Journal of Arthroplasty, 18(1),* 69–74.

Lin JJ, Kaplan RJ (2004) Multivariate analysis of the factors affecting duration of acute inpatient rehabilitation after hip and knee arthroplasty. *American Journal of Physical Medicine and Rehabilitation, 83(5),* 344–352.

Malik MH, Lovell ME, Jones M (2002) Patient-related factors leading to total hip replacement dislocation: a case series. *Advances in Physiotherapy, 4(2),* 85–86.

Malviya A, Wilson G, Kleim B, Kurtz AM, Deehan D (2014) Factors influencing return to work after hip and knee replacement. *Occupational Medicine, 64(6)*, 402–409.

Mancuso CA, Sculco TP, Salvati EA (2003) Patients with poor pre-operative functional status have high expectations of total hip arthroplasty. *The Journal of Arthroplasty, 18(7)*, 872–878.

Marks R (2008) Hip surgery candidates: a comparative study of hip osteoarthritis and prior hip fracture patient characteristics. [Online] *The Open Orthopaedics Journal, 2*, 79–85. Available at: *https://www.ncbi.nlm.nih.gov/pmc/articles/PMC2687111/pdf/TOORTHJ-2-79.pdf*

McDonald S, Hetrick SE, Green S (2004) (1) *Pre-operative education for hip or knee replacement*. (Cochrane Review). Chichester, UK: John Wiley & Sons, Ltd. Available at: *http://onlinelibrary.wiley.com/doi/10.1002/14651858.CD003526.pub2/full*

McDonald S, Page MJ, Beringer K, Wasiak J, Sprowson A (2014) *Preoperative education for hip or knee replacement.* (Cochrane Review). Chichester, UK: John Wiley & Sons, Ltd. Available at: *http://www.cochrane.org/CD003526/MUSKEL_preoperative-education-hip-or-knee-replacement*

McHugh G, Luker K (2012) Individuals' expectations and challenges following total hip replacement: a qualitative study. *Disability and Rehabilitation, 34(16)*, 1351–1357.

McQuaid L, Cope J, Fenech A (2014) Occupational therapy in orthopaedics: an alternative to hip precautions? [Online] *International Journal of Therapy and Rehabilitation, 21(11)*, 508–510. Available at: *http://dx.doi.org/10.12968/ijtr.2014.21.11.508*

Mobasheri R, Gidwani S, Rosson JW (2006) The effect of total hip replacement on the employment status of patients under the age of 60 years. *Annals of the Royal College of Surgeons of England, 88(2)*, 131–133.

Montin L, Leino-Kilpi H, Katajisto J, Lepistö J, Kettunen J, Suominen T (2007) Anxiety and health-related quality of life of patients undergoing total hip arthroplasty for osteoarthritis. *Chronic Illness, 3(3)*, 219–227.

Naylor JM, Harmer AR, Heard RC (2008) Severe other joint disease and obesity independently influence recovery after joint replacement surgery: an observational study. *Australian Journal of Physiotherapy, 54(1)*, 57–64.

Nickinson RS, Board TN, Kay PR (2009) Post-operative anxiety and depression levels in orthopaedics surgery: a study of 56 patients undergoing hip or knee arthroplasty. *Journal of Evaluation in Clinical Practice, 15(2)*, 307–310.

Nunley RM, Ruh EL, Zhang Q, Della Valle CJ, Engh Jr CA, Berend E. . .Barrack RL (2011) Do patients return to work after hip arthroplasty surgery? *The Journal of Arthroplasty, 26* (*6, Supplement*), 92–98.e3.

Oberg T, Oberg U, Sviden G, Persson AN (2005) Functional capacity after hip arthroplasty: a comparison between evaluation with three standard instruments and a personal interview. *Scandinavian Journal of Occupational Therapy, 12(1)*, 18–28.

O'Donnell S, Kennedy D, MacLeod AM, Kilroy C, Gollish J (2006) Achieving team consensus on best practice rehabilitation guidelines following primary total hip replacement (THR) surgery. *Healthcare Quarterly, 9(4),* 60–64.

Ollivier M, Frey S, Parratte S, Flecher X, Argenson JN (2014) Pre-operative function, motivation and duration of symptoms predict sporting participation after total hip replacement. *The Bone and Joint Journal, 96-B(8),* 1041–1046.

Orpen N, Harris J (2010) Patients' perceptions of pre-operative home-based occupational therapy and/or physiotherapy interventions prior to total hip replacement. *British Journal of Occupational Therapy, 73(10),* 461–469.

Ostendorf M, van Stel HF, Buskens E, Schrijvers AJ, Marting LN, Verbout AJ, Dhert WJ (2004) Patient-reported outcome in total hip replacement: a comparison of five instruments of health status. *The Journal of Bone & Joint Surgery* (British Volume), *86-B(6),* 801–808.

Pape B, Thiessen PS, Jakobsen F, Hansen TB (2013) Interprofessional collaboration may pay off: introducing a collaborative approach in an orthopaedic ward. *Journal of Interprofessional Care, 27(6),* 496–500.

Parsons GE, Godfrey H, Jester RF (2009) Living with severe osteoarthritis while awaiting hip and knee joint replacement surgery. *Musculoskeletal Care, 7(2),* 121–135.

Peak EL, Parvizi J, Ciminiello M, Purtill JJ, Sharkey PF, Hozack WJ, Rothman RH (2005) The role of patient restrictions in reducing the prevalence of early dislocation following total hip arthroplasty: a randomised, prospective study. *The Journal of Bone & Joint Surgery (American Volume), 87(2),* 247–253.

Restrepo C, Mortazavi SMJ, Brothers B, Parvizi J, Rothman R (2011) Hip dislocation: are hip precautions necessary in anterior approaches? *Clinical Orthopaedics and Related Research, 469(2),* 417–422.

Rivard A, Warren S, Voaklander D, Jones A (2003) The efficacy of pre-operative home visits for total hip replacement clients. *Canadian Journal of Occupational Therapy, 70(4),* 226–232.

Sankar A, Davis AM, Palaganas MP, Beaton DE, Badley EM, Gignac MA (2013) Return to work and workplace activity limitations following total hip or knee replacement. *Osteoarthritis and Cartilage, 21(10),* 1485–1493.

Siggeirsdottir K, Olafsson O, Jonsson Jr H, Iwarsson S, Gudnason V, Jonsson BY (2005) Short hospital stay augmented with education and home-based rehabilitation improves function and quality of life after hip replacement: randomised study of 50 patients with 6 months of follow-up. *Acta Orthopaedicsa, 76(4),* 555–562.

Smith TO, Jepson P, Beswick A, Sands G, Drummond A, Davis ET, Sackley CM (2016) *Assistive devices, hip precautions, environmental modifications and training to prevent dislocation and improve function after hip arthroplasty.* (Cochrane Review). Chichester, UK: John Wiley & Sons, Ltd. Available at: *http://onlinelibrary.wiley.com/doi/10.1002/14651858.CD010815.pub2/full*

Smith TO, Sackley CM (2016) UK survey of occupational therapist's and physiotherapist's experiences and attitudes towards hip replacement precautions and equipment. [Online] *BMC Musculoskeletal Disorders, 17(228)*. Available at: *https://bmcmusculoskeletdisord.biomedcentral.com/articles/10.1186/s12891-016-1092-x*

Smith T, Latham S, Maskrey V, Blyth A (2015) Patients' perceptions of physical activity before and after joint replacement: a systematic review with meta-ethnographic analysis. *Postgraduate Medical Journal, 91(1079),* 483–491.

Soever LJ, MacKay C, Saryeddine T, Davis AM, Flannery JF, Jaglal SB. . .Mahomed N (2010) Educational needs of patients undergoing total joint arthroplasty. *Physiotherapy Canada, 62(3),* 206–214.

Spalding NJ (2004) Pre-operative education: empowering patients with confidence. *International Journal of Therapy and Rehabilitation, 11(4),* 147–153.

Spalding NJ (2003) Reducing anxiety by pre-operative education: make the future familiar. *Occupational Therapy International, 10(4),* 278–293.

Stewart LSP, McMillan IR (2011) How necessary are hip restrictions for avoiding dislocation following hemiarthroplasty or total hip arthroplasty in older patients with a hip fracture? *British Journal of Occupational Therapy, 74(3),* 110–118.

Thomas WN, Pinkelman LA, Gardine CJ (2010) The reasons for noncompliance with adaptive equipment in patients returning home after a total hip replacement. *Physical & Occupational Therapy in Geriatrics, 28(2),* 170–180.

van der Weegen W, Kornuijt A, Das D (2016) Do lifestyle restrictions and precautions prevent dislocation after total hip arthroplasty? A systematic review and meta-analysis of the literature. *Clinical Rehabilitation, 30(4),* 329–339.

Ververeli PA, Lebby EB, Tyler C, Fouad C (2009) Evaluation of reducing post-operative hip precautions in total hip replacement: a randomised prospective study. *Orthopedics, 32(12),* 889–893.

Vincent H, Horodyski MB, Gearen P, Vlasak R, Seay A, Conrad B, Vincent K (2012) Obesity and long term functional outcomes following elective total hip replacement. [Online]. *Journal of Orthopaedic Surgery and Research, 7(16)*. Available at: *http://www.josr-online.com/content/7/1/16*

Vincent HK, Weng JP, Vincent KR (2007) Effect of obesity on inpatient rehabilitation outcomes after total hip arthroplasty. *Obesity (Silver Spring), 15(2),* 522–530.

Vissers MM, Bussmann BJ, de Groot IB, Verhaar JAN, Reijman M (2013) Physical functioning four years after total hip and knee arthroplasty. *Gait and Posture, 38(2),* 310–315.

Wagenmakers R, Stevens M, Groothoff JW, Zijlstra W, Bulstra SK, van Beveren J. . .van den Akker-Scheek I (2011) Physical activity behavior of patients one year after primary total hip arthroplasty: a prospective multicenter cohort study. *Physical Therapy, 91(3),* 373–380.

Wang W, Morrison TA, Geller JA, Yoon RS, Macaulay W (2010) Predicting short-term outcome of primary total hip arthroplasty: a prospective multivariate regression analysis of 12 independent factors. *The Journal of Arthroplasty, 25(6),* 858–864.

Wang X, Emery LJ (2002) Cognitive status after hip replacement. *Physical & Occupational Therapy in Geriatrics, 21(1),* 51–64.

Williams DH, Greidanus NV, Masri BA, Duncan CP, Garbuz DS (2012) Predictors of participation in sports after hip and knee arthroplasty. *Clinical Orthopaedics and Related Research, 470(2),* 555–561.

Wilson MJ, Villar RN (2011) Hip replacement in the athlete: is there a role? *Knee surgery, Sports Traumatology, Arthroscopy, 19(9),* 1524–1530.

Wong J, Wong S, Brooks E (2002) A study of hospital recovery pattern of acutely confused older patients following hip surgery. *International Journal of Orthopaedic and Trauma Nursing, 6(2),* 68–78.

Supporting information references

Blom A, Rogers M, Taylor A, Pattison G, Whitehouse S, Bannister G (2008) Dislocation following total hip replacement: the Avon Orthopaedics Centre experience. *Annals of the Royal College of Surgeons England, 90(8),* 658–662.

British Orthopaedic Association (2012) *Primary total hip replacement: a guide to good practice.* London: BOA. Available at: *https://www.britishhipsociety.com/uploaded/Blue%20Book%202012%20fsh%20nov%202012.pdf*

British Orthopaedic Association (2006) *Primary total hip replacement: a guide to good practice*. London: BOA.

College of Occupational Therapists (2017a) *Practice guideline development manual.* 3rd ed. London: COT. Available at: *https://www.rcot.co.uk/sites/default/files/Practice-guidelines-development-manual-Third-edition.pdf*

College of Occupational Therapists (2017b) *Professional standards for occupational therapy practice.* London: COT. Available at: *https://www.rcot.co.uk/practice-resources/rcot-publications/downloads/rcot-standards-and-ethics*

College of Occupational Therapists (2016) *What is occupational therapy?* London: COT. Available at: *https://www.rcot.co.uk/about-occupational-therapy/what-is-occupational-therapy*

College of Occupational Therapists (2015a) *Occupational therapy in the prevention and management of falls in adults: practice guideline.* London: COT. Available at: *https://www.rcot.co.uk/practice-resources/rcot-publications/member/practice-guidelines-publications*

College of Occupational Therapists (2015b) *Code of ethics and professional conduct.* London: COT. Available at: *https://www.rcot.co.uk/practice-resources/rcot-publications/downloads/rcot-standards-and-ethics*

College of Occupational Therapists (2011) *Practice guidelines development manual.* 2nd ed. London: COT.

College of Occupational Therapists (2007) *Building the evidence for occupational therapy: priorities for research.* London: COT. Available at: *https://www.rcot.co.uk/practice-resources/rcot-publications/member/research-and-review-publications*

College of Occupational Therapists and National Social Inclusion Programme (2007) *Work matters: vocational navigation for occupational therapy staff.* London: COT/NSIP. Available at: *https://www.rcot.co.uk/practice-resources/rcot-publications/member/guidance*

Coole C, Nouri F, Drummond A (2016) The rise and rise of hip and knee replacement. *OTnews, 24(12)*, 28–29.

Critical Appraisal Skills Programme (2010) *CASP checklists.* Available at: *http://www.casp-uk.net/*

Culliford D, Maskell J, Judge A, Cooper C, Prieto-Alhambra D, Arden NK (2015) Future projections of total hip and knee arthroplasty in the UK: results from the UK Clinical Practice Research Datalink. *Osteoarthritis and Cartilage 23(4)*, 594–600.

Department of Health (2006) *The musculoskeletal services framework a joint responsibility: doing it differently*. London: DH. Available at: *http://webarchive.nationalarchives.gov.uk/20130124073659/http://www.dh.gov.uk/prod_consum_dh/groups/dh_digitalassets/@dh/@en/documents/digitalasset/dh_4138412.pdf*

GRADE Working Group (2004) Grading quality of evidence and strength of recommendations. *British Medical Journal, 328(7454)*, 1490–1494.

Gustafsson BÅ, Ekman SL, Ponzer S, Heikkilä K (2010) The hip and knee replacement operation: an extensive life event. *Scandinavian Journal of Caring Sciences, 24(4)*, 663–670.

Guyatt GH, Oxman AD, Kunz R, Falck-Ytter Y, Vist GE, Liberati A. . .GRADE working Group (2008) Rating quality of evidence and strength of recommendations: going from evidence to recommendations. *British Medical Journal, 336(7652)*, 1049–1051.

Harte D, Hamill P, Williams-Condell C, Lewis S (2017) Evaluation of the impact of preoperative assessment on length of stay after a total hip arthroplasty. [Online]. *British Journal of Occupational Therapy, 80(6)*, 361–367.

Health and Care Professions Council (2016a) *Number of OTs: August 2016*. London: HCPC. Available at: *http://www.hcpc-uk.org/publications/foi/index.asp?id=1253*

Health and Care Professions Council (2016b) *Standards of conduct, performance and ethics.* London: HCPC. Available at: *http://www.hcpc-uk.org/publications/standards/index.asp?id=38*

Health and Care Professions Council (2013) *Standards of proficiency: occupational therapists.* London: HCPC. Available at: *http://www.hcpc-uk.org/publications/standards/index.asp?id=45*

Marmot M, Allen J, Goldblatt P, Boyce T, McNeish D, Grady M, Geddes I (2010) *Fair society, healthy lives: the Marmot review.* [London]: Marmot Review. Available at: *http://www.instituteofhealthequity.org/resources-reports/fair-society-healthy-lives-the-marmot-review/fair-society-healthy-lives-full-report-pdf.pdf*

Monitor, NHS England (2016a) *[2016/17 national tariff payment system]: annex A: 2016/17 national prices and national tariff workbook*. London: Monitor. Available at: *https://www.gov.uk/government/publications/nhs-national-tariff-payment-system-201617*

Monitor, NHS England (2016b) [2016/17 *national tariff payment system]: annex B: technical guidance and information for services with national currencies.* London: Monitor. Available at: *https://www.gov.uk/government/publications/nhs-national-tariff-payment-system-201617*

National Audit Office (2003) *Hip replacements: an update.* London: The Stationery Office.

National Institute for Health and Care Excellence (2017) *Musculoskeletal conditions overview.* London: NICE. Available at: *https://pathways.nice.org.uk/pathways/musculoskeletal-conditions*

National Institute for Health and Care Excellence (2014) *Osteoarthritis: care and management.* (Clinical Guideline CG177). London: NICE. Available at: *https://www.nice.org.uk/guidance/cg177/resources/osteoarthritis-care-and-management-35109757272517*

National Institute for Health and Care Excellence (2013) *Falls in older people: assessing risk and prevention.* (Clinical Guideline CG161). London: NICE. Available at: *https://www.nice.org.uk/guidance/cg161/resources/falls-in-older-people-assessing-risk-and-prevention-35109686728645*

National Institute for Health and Care Excellence (2012) *Hip fracture for adults: quality standard*. (QS16). London: NICE. (Last updated 2014). Available at: *https://www.nice.org.uk/guidance/qs16/resources/hip-fracture-in-adults-pdf-2098488670405*

National Institute for Health and Care Excellence (2011) *Hip fracture: management.* (Clinical Guideline CG124). London: NICE. (Last updated 2014). Available at: *https://www.nice.org.uk/guidance/cg124/resources/hip-fracture-management-pdf-35109449902789*

National Joint Registry (2016) *National Joint Registry for England, Wales, Northern Ireland and the Isle of Man: 13th annual report 2016.* Hemel Hempstead: NJR. Available at: *http://www.njrreports.org.uk/Portals/0/PDFdownloads/NJR%2013th%20Annual%20Report%202016.pdf*

National Joint Registry (2011) *National Joint Registry for England and Wales: 8th annual report 2011*. Hemel Hempstead: NJR. Available at: *http://www.njrcentre.org.uk/njrcentre/Portals/0/Documents/NJR%208th%20Annual%20Report%202011.pdf*

NHS Digital (2017) *Patient Reported Outcome Measures (PROMs)*. Leeds: NHS Digital. Available at: *http://content.digital.nhs.uk/proms*

NHS Digital (2015) *Hospital episode Statistics, admitted patient care: England, 2014–15 [NS].* Leeds: NHS Digital. Available at: *http://content.digital.nhs.uk/catalogue/PUB19124*

NHS National Services Scotland (2016) *Scottish arthroplasty project: biennial report 2016*. Edinburgh: NHS National Services Scotland. Available at: *http://www.arthro.scot.nhs.uk/docs/2016-08-09-SAP-Report.pdf?1*

NHS National Services Scotland (2010) *Scottish arthroplasty project: annual report 2010*. Edinburgh: NHS National Services Scotland. Available at: *http://www.arthro.scot.nhs.uk/Scottish_Arthroplasty_Project_Report_2010.pdf*

NHS South East Coast (2012) *Orthopaedics enhanced recovery programme: to reduce length of hospital stay*. (11/0041 QIPP Collection). London: NICE. Originally sourced from: *https://www.nice.org.uk/about/what-we-do/into-practice/local-practice-case-studies.* [No longer available]

Richardson WS, Wilson MC, Nishikawa J, Hayward RS (1995) The well-built clinical question: a key to evidence-based decisions. *ACP Journal Club, 123(3)*, A12–13.

Royal College of Surgeons of England; British Orthopaedic Association (2000) *National total hip replacement outcome study: final report to the Department of Health.* London: Royal College of Surgeons of England.

Scottish Intercollegiate Guidelines Network (2009) *Management of hip fracture in older people: a national clinical guideline: [number] 111).* Edinburgh: SIGN.

Wales Audit Office (2015) *A review of orthopaedic services.* Cardiff: Wales Audit Office. Available at: *http://www.audit.wales/system/files/publications/Review_of_orthopaedic_ENG%20_2015.pdf*

World Federation of Occupational Therapists (2013) *Definitions of occupational therapy from member organisations.* Forrestfield, AU: WFOT. (This document can be accessed from the Resource Centre, filter resources by category: 'General'). Available at: *http://wfot.org/resourcecentre.aspx*

Worrall M (2010) Many small steps to reducing length of stay: a visit to the DH pilot enhanced recovery scheme. *The Bulletin of the Royal College of Surgeons of England, 92(8)*, 266–268.

All websites in these references were accessed on 26.07.17